a **CORE**
Curriculum
for Diabetes
Education
Fifth Edition

Diabetes
and
Complications

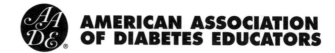

AMERICAN ASSOCIATION
OF DIABETES EDUCATORS

a **CORE**
Curriculum
for Diabetes
Education
Fifth Edition

Diabetes and Complications

Editor
Marion J. Franz, MS, RD, LD, CDE

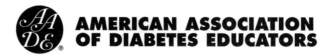

**AMERICAN ASSOCIATION
OF DIABETES EDUCATORS**

a CORE Curriculum for Diabetes Education, 5th Edition
Diabetes and Complications
Published by the American Association of Diabetes Educators

©2003, American Association of Diabetes Educators, Chicago, Illinois.
ISBN 1-881876-11-X (Volume One)
ISBN 1-881876-15-2 (Four-Volume Set)

Library of Congress Control Number: 2003108781

Printed and bound in the United States of America.

a CORE Curriculum for Diabetes Education

Diabetes and Complications

In this Volume:

Table of Contents

Diabetes and Complications

Introduction/Acknowledgements

It is an exciting and challenging time for diabetes education. Exciting because of the many advances that help people better manage their diabetes—new medications, technologies, research that makes lifestyle recommendations easier to understand and apply, the empowerment approach to education, to name just a few. The challenges and frustrations are the difficulties of sharing this information with individuals with diabetes, the lack of opportunities to individualize care, and the lack of time to assist in facilitating behavior changes. Resources—personnel, payment for services, maintaining education centers—are other challenges. The CORE Curriculum cannot solve all the challenges, but it can update healthcare providers' knowledge and skills and provide suggestions for facilitating behavior changes in persons with diabetes.

The CORE Curriculum was originally planned to help educators prepare for the Certified Diabetes Educator (CDE) exam. This has continued to be a goal for subsequent editions; however, the use and the scope of the CORE Curriculum has expanded. It is a key reference for the Advanced Diabetes Management credential exam. The CORE Curriculum has also evolved into being an authoritative source of information for diabetes education, training, and management. Just as all medicine is moving toward evidence-based practice, this must also be a goal for education. Chapters must have appropriate and adequate references, and as a reader you have the right to question statements in the CORE Curriculum that do not have adequate documentation. Continuing this focus will result in the CORE Curriculum becoming more evidence-based. Another goal is to have the CORE Curriculum reflect a team approach to education and management. It is exciting to see the number of management chapters written by a team of healthcare providers.

As with all projects of this size, there are many individuals to whom we are indebted. It begins with the chapter authors, who are willing to share their expertise and provide up-to-date information and management skills for the reader. It continues to the chapter reviewers, who provide suggestions to make the chapters stronger. The authors and reviewers are listed in each volume of the CORE Curriculum. When you see these individuals, please extend your thanks to them for the valuable service they provide. The Editorial Board—Janine Freeman, Barbara McCloskey, Charlotte Nath, and William Polonsky—provide suggestions to improve the CORE Curriculum and valuable reviewer assistance. Dr. Lois Book, RN, Director of Professional Relations, at the AADE National Office provides valuable suggestions for CORE content and support for the process of writing and editing of the CORE Curriculum. We are fortunate to work with very competent editorial and publishing professionals. Mary Beach at Stenson Bauer Communications keeps the process moving efficiently. Nancy Williams uses her copyreader and editing skills to make sure small details and mistakes are not missed. Karen Lloyd provides editorial assistance for the new chapters, and Michele Montour at Montronics makes sure text is accurately typeset. To all these important professionals, the AADE owes a great deal of gratitude.

The CORE Curriculum would not be possible without the contributions of previous editors—Diana Guthrie, Julie Meyer, Kathryn Godley, Virginia Peragallo-Dittko, and Martha Funnell. Each edition moved the professionalism of the CORE Curriculum forward, and those who worked on this edition sincerely hope to have continued that tradition. As authors, reviewers, and editors, we have done our best to make this edition a valuable resource for all diabetes educators and healthcare providers. We welcome suggestions from you as you read and use the CORE Curriculum as to how it can become a better and more useful resource. Please use the CORE Curriculum to improve the education and care that you provide for people with diabetes. That ultimately is the final goal, to enrich the lives of persons with diabetes who have been, for all of us, our best educators!

Marion J. Franz, MS, RD, LD, CDE
Editor, CORE Curriculum, 5th Edition

Editor

Marion J. Franz, MS, RD, LD, CDE
Nutrition Concepts by Franz, Inc.
Minneapolis, Minnesota

Associate Editors

Karmeen Kulkarni, MS, RD, BC-ADM, CDE
St. Marks Hospital Diabetes Center
Salt Lake City, Utah

William H. Polonsky, PhD, CDE
Department of Psychiatry
University of California
San Diego, California

Peggy Yarborough, MS, RPh, BC-ADM, CDE
Campbell University and Wilson Community Health Center
Wilson, North Carolina

Virginia Zamudio, RN, MSN, CDE
Alamo Diabetes Team
San Antonio, Texas

Authors

Jessie H. Ahroni,
PhD, ARNP, CDE
Veterans Affairs Puget Sound
Health Care System
School of Nursing, University
of Washington
Seattle, Washington

Robert M. Anderson, EdD
Michigan Diabetes Research
and Training Center
University of Michigan
Ann Arbor, Michigan

James D. Anderst, MD
Medical College of Wisconsin
Milwaukee, Wisconsin

Mindy Andrus,
RD, LDN, CDE
East Carolina University
Brody School of Medicine
Greenville, North Carolina

Susan L. Barlow, RD, CDE
Amylin Pharmaceuticals, Inc.
Indianapolis, Indiana

Marla Bernbaum, MD
St. Louis University Health
Sciences Center
Division of Endocrinology
St. Louis, Missouri

Jean Betschart,
MSN, MN, CPNP, CDE
Children's Hospital
of Pittsburgh
Pittsburgh, Pennsylvania

Susan A. Biastre,
RD, LDN, CDE
Women & Infants' Hospital
Providence, Rhode Island

Ann Marie Brooks, RN, CDE
St. Marks Hospital
Diabetes Center
Salt Lake City, Utah

R. Keith Campbell,
RPh, MBA, CDE
Washington State University
Spokane, Washington

Belinda P. Childs, RN, MN,
ARNP, CDE
Mid-America Diabetes
Associates
Wichita, Kansas

Beth Ann Coonrod, PhD,
MPH, RN, CDE
Heritage Valley Health
System
Beaver and Sewickley,
Pennsylvania

Angela D'Antonio, RD
University of South Carolina
Norman J. Arnold School of
Public Health
Columbia, South Carolina

Mayer B. Davidson, MD
Charles R. Drew University
Los Angeles, California

Kristina L. Ernst,
BSN, RN, CDE
Atlanta, Georgia

James A. Fain,
PhD, RN, FAAN
University of Massachusetts
Worcester
Graduate School of Nursing
Worcester, Massachusetts

Eva L. Feldman, MD, PhD
Department of Neurology
University of Michigan
Medical School
Ann Arbor, Michigan

Marion J. Franz,
MS, RD, LD, CDE
Nutrition Concepts
by Franz, Inc.
Minneapolis, Minnesota

Martha Mitchell Funnell,
MS, RN, CDE
Michigan Diabetes Research
and Training Center
University of Michigan
Medical Center
Ann Arbor, Michigan

Patti Geil, MS, RD, CDE
Lexington, Kentucky

Linda Gonder-Frederick, PhD
University of Virginia
Behavioral Medicine Center
Charlottesville, Virginia

Diana W. Guthrie,
RN, ARNP, FAAN, CDE
Professor Emeritus
University of Kansas School
of Medicine
Wichita, Kansas

Richard A. Guthrie,
MD, CDE
Mid-America Diabetes
Associates
Via Christi Regional
Medical Center
University of Kansas School
of Medicine
Wichita, Kansas

Deborah Hinnen,
RN, MN, ARNP,
BC-ADM, CDE
Via Christi Regional
Medical Center
Wichita, Kansas

Carol Homko,
RN, PhD, CDE
Temple University Hospital
Philadelphia, Pennsylvania

Cheryl Hunt,
RN, MSEd, CDE
Health Education
and Resources
Alexandria, Virginia

Donna Jornsay,
BSN, RN, CPNP, CDE
MiniMed
Great Neck, New York

Elaine Boswell King,
MSN, RN, CS, CDE
Vanderbilt Diabetes Research
and Training Center
Nashville, Tennessee

Karmeen Kulkarni,
MS, RD, BC-ADM, CDE
St. Marks Hospital
Diabetes Center
Salt Lake City, Utah

Janie Lipps,
MSN, RN, CS, CDE
Vanderbilt Diabetes Research
and Training Center
Nashville, Tennessee

Nancy Leggett-Frazier,
RN, MSN, CDE
East Carolina University
Brody School of Medicine
Greenville, North Carolina

Elizabeth J. Mayer-Davis,
PhD, RD
University of South Carolina
Norman J. Arnold School of
Public Health
Columbia, South Carolina

Stephania Miller, PhD
Diabetes Research and
Training Center
Vanderbilt University
School of Medicine
Nashville, Tennessee

Catherine A. Mullooly,
MS, RCEPsм, CDE
Joslin Clinic
Boston, Massachusetts

Kathryn Mulcahy,
RN, MSN, CDE
Fairfax Hospital INOVA
Diabetes Center
Fairfax, Virginia

Joseph P. Napora,
PhD, LCSW-C
The Johns Hopkins
University School of Medicine
The Johns Hopkins
Diabetes Center
Baltimore, Maryland

Anne T. Nettles,
RN, MS, CDE
Healthcare Consultant
Minneapolis, Minnesota

Jan Norman, RD, CDE
Washington Department
of Health
Diabetes Control Program
Olympia, Washington

Virginia Peragallo-Dittko,
RN, MA, CDE
Diabetes Education Center
Winthrop-University Hospital
Mineola, New York

Michael A. Pfeifer,
MD, FACE, CDE
East Carolina University
Brody School of Medicine
Greenville, North Carolina

James W. Pichert, PhD
Diabetes Research and
Training Center
Vanderbilt University
Nashville, Tennessee

Robert E. Ratner, MD, CDE
Medstar Research Institute
Washington, DC

Lynne S. Robbins, PhD
University of Washington
Department of
Medical Education
Seattle, Washington

Richard R. Rubin, PhD, CDE
The Johns Hopkins
University School of Medicine
Departments of Medicine
and Pediatrics
Baltimore, Maryland

Stephanie Schwartz,
MPH, RN, CDE
Children With Diabetes .Com
Ann Arbor, Michigan

Laura Shane-McWhorter,
PharmD, BCPS, FASCP, CDE
College of Pharmacy
University of Utah
Salt Lake City, Utah

Tamara Stich,
RN, MSN, CDE
Washington University School
of Medicine
Department of Metabolism
St. Louis, Missouri

Catrine Tudor-Locke, PhD
University of South Carolina
Norman J. Arnold School of
Public Health
Columbia, South Carolina

Frank Vinicor, MD, MPH
Centers for Disease
Control and Prevention
Division of Diabetes
Translation
Atlanta, Georgia

John R. White, Jr.,
RPh, PharmD, PA-C
Washington State University
Spokane, Washington

Peggy C. Yarborough,
RPh, MS, BC-ADM, CDE
Campbell University and
Wilson Community
Health Center
Wilson, North Carolina

Reviewers

Barbara J. Anderson, PhD
Joslin Diabetes Center
Harvard University School
of Medicine
Boston, Massachusetts

Gary M. Arsham, MD, PhD
Arsham Consultants, Inc.
San Francisco, California

Anita K. Austin, RPh, CDE
University of Pittsburgh
Physicians
Pittsburgh, Pennsylvania

David W. Bartels,
PharmD, CDE
University of Illinois at
Chicago College of Pharmacy
Department of Pharmacy
Practice and College of
Medicine at Rockford
Department of Family and
Community Medicine

David S. Bell, MD
University of Alabama
Medical School
Birmingham, Alabama

Kathy J. Berkowitz,
RNC, FNP, CDE
Diabetes Unit, Grady
Health System
Atlanta, Georgia

Liz Blair, ANP, CDE
Joslin Diabetes Center
Boston, Massachusetts

Barbara H. Bodnar,
RN, MS, CDE
West Virginia University
Morgantown, West Virginia

John B. Buse, MD, PhD, CDE
University of North Carolina
Diabetes Care Center
Durham, North Carolina

Denise Charron-Prochownik,
PhD, RN, CPNP
University of Pittsburgh
School of Nursing/
Health Promotion
Pittsburgh, Pennsylvania

Belinda Childs, RN, MN,
ARNP, CDE
Mid-America Diabetes
Associates, PA
Wichita, Kansas

Beth Ann Coonrod,
PhD, MPH, RN, CDE
Heritage Valley Health
System
Beaver and Sewickley,
Pennsylvania

Alicia Correa,
RN, BSN, MBA
Texas Diabetes Institute
San Antonio, Texas

Marjorie Cypress,
MSN, C-ANP, CDE
Lovelace Medical Center
Endocrinology/Diabetes
Department
Albuquerque, New Mexico

Anne Daly,
MS, RD, LD, BC-ADM, CDE
Springfield Diabetes and
Endocrine Center
Springfield, Illinois

Mary Ellinger, RD, CDE
Diabetes Self Care,
Matria Healthcare
Centreville, Virginia

Janine Freeman,
RD, LD, CDE
Diabetes Nutrition Specialist
Atlanta, Georgia

Sandra J. Gillespie,
MMSc, RD, LD, CDE
Diabetes Resource Center
Piedmont Hospital
Atlanta, Georgia

Russell E. Glasgow, PhD
AMC Cancer Research
Center
Denver, Colorado

Kathryn Godley,
MS, RN, CDE
Albany Medical College
Albany, New York

Marilyn R. Graff,
RN, BSN, CDE
MiniMed Professional
Education Department
Sylmar, California

Richard A. Guthrie,
MD, FCAP, CDE
Mid-America Diabetes
Associates, Inc.
Wichita, Kansas

Leo E. Hendricks,
PhD, LICSW, CDE
LHCA's Diabetes Self-
Management Skills
Training Center
Silver Springs, Maryland

Rosetta T. Hendricks,
PhD, RN, CS, FNP, CDE
Veterans Affairs
Medical Center
Washington, DC

Lea Ann Holzmeister,
RD, CDE
Nutrition Consultant
Tempe, Arizona

David Holtzman
Director of
Government Affairs
American Association of
Diabetes Educators
Chicago, Illinois

Bonnie Irvin,
MS, RD, LD, CDE
Iredell Memorial Hospital
Health Care System
Diabetes Center for Learning
Statesville, North Carolina

Timothy J. Ives,
PharmD, MPH
Department of
Family Medicine
University of North Carolina
Chapel Hill, North Carolina

Scott J. Jacober, DO, CDE
Eli Lilly & Co.
Indianapolis, Indiana

Dennis Janisse, CPed
National Pedorthic Services
Milwaukee, Wisconsin

Jane Kadohiro,
DrPH, APRN, CDE
University of Hawaii School
of Nursing and
Dental Hygiene
Honolulu, Hawaii

Ginger Kanzer-Lewis,
RNC, EdM, CDE
GKL Associates
Pomona, New York

Wahida Karmally,
MS, RD, CDE
The Irving Center for Clinical
Research, Columbia
University
New York, New York

Julienne K. Kirk,
PharmD, CDE, BCPS
Department of Family
Medicine
Wake Forest University
School of Medicine
Winston-Salem,
North Carolina

Davida F. Kruger,
MSN, RN, BC-ADM, CDE
Henry Ford Health Systems
Endocrinology/Metabolism
Detroit, Michigan

Andrea J. Lasichak,
MS, RD, CDE
Michigan Diabetes Research
Training Center
University of
Michigan Hospital
Ann Arbor, Michigan

Daniel Lorber,
MD, FACP, CDE
Diabetes Control Foundation
Flushing, New York

Melinda D. Maryniuk,
MEd, RD, FADA, CDE
Joslin Diabetes Center
Boston, Massachusetts

Susan McLaughlin, RD, CDE
On-Site Health &
Wellness, LLC
Omaha, Nebraska

Arlene Monk, RD, LD, CDE
International Diabetes Center
Minneapolis, Minnesota

Arshag D. Mooradian, MD
St. Louis University Medical
Center Division of
Endocrinology
St. Louis, Missouri

Charlotte Reese Nath,
MSN, RN, EdD, CDE
West Virginia University
Department of Family
Medicine
Robert C. Byrd Health
Sciences Center
Morgantown, West Virginia

Jan Nicollerat,
MSN, RN, CS, CDE
Duke University Adult
Diabetes Education Program
Cary, North Carolina

Jan Norman, RD, CD, CDE
Washington State
Department of Health
Olympia, Washington

Belinda O'Connell,
MS, RD, CDE
International Diabetes Center
Minneapolis, Minnesota

Joyce G. Pastors,
RD, MS, CDE
Virginia Center for Diabetes
Professional Education
Charlottesville, Virginia

Teresa L. Pearson,
MS, RN, CDE
Health Partners Center for
Health Promotion
Minneapolis, Minnesota

Suzanne Pecoraro,
RD, MPH, CDE
Diabetes Education Society
Denver, Colorado

Martha Price,
DNSc, ARNP, CDE
Group Health Cooperative
Diabetes Clinical Roadmap
Seattle, Washington

Diane M. Reader, RD, CDE
International Diabetes Center
Minneapolis, Minnesota

Dawn Satterfield,
RNC, MSN, CDE
Centers for Disease Control
and Prevention
Division of Diabetes
Translation
Atlanta, Georgia

J. Terry Saunders, PhD
Virginia Center for Diabetes
Professional Education
Charlottesville, Virginia

Pamela Scarborough,
PT, MS, CDE, CWS
Education 2000 Plus
Dallas, Texas

Gary Scheiner, MS, CDE
Integrated Diabetes Services
Wynnewood, Pennsylvania

Barbara Schreiner,
RN, MN, BC-ADM, CDE
Texas Children's Hospital
Diabetes Care Center
Houston, Texas

Michelle Burdette-Taylor
BT & T Health Education
with a Purpose
San Diego, California

Christine Tobin,
RN, MBA, CDE
Health Care Consultant
Atlanta, Georgia

Elizabeth A. Walker,
RN, DNSc, CDE
Albert Einstein College
of Medicine
Diabetes Research and
Training Center
Bronx, New York

Hope S. Warshaw,
MMSc, RD, CDE
Hope Warshaw Associates
Alexandria, Virginia

Madelyn L. Wheeler,
MS, RD, FADA, CDE
Diabetes Research and
Training Center
Indiana University School
of Medicine
Indianapolis, Indiana

Neil H. White, MD, CDE
Pediatric Endocrinology and
Metabolism
Washington University
St. Louis, Missouri

Ann Sawyer Williams,
MSN, RN, CDE
Cleveland Heights, Ohio

Donald N. Zettervall,
RPH, CDE
The Diabetes Center
Old Saybrook, Connecticut

A Core Curriculum for Diabetes Education
Diabetes and Complications

Pathophysiology of the Diabetes Disease State   1

Robert E. Ratner, MD, CDE
Medstar Research Institute
Washington, DC

Introduction

1 Diabetes mellitus is sometimes described by both patients and health professionals as "a little bit of sugar" or "high sugar." In reality, "sugar" is only one component of the pathology and clinical manifestations of the multifaceted syndrome of diabetes mellitus.

2 Diabetes mellitus may be broadly described as a chronic, systemic disease characterized by

A Abnormalities in the metabolism of carbohydrates, proteins, fats, and insulin

B Abnormalities in the structure and function of blood vessels and nerves

3 The pathophysiology leading to the development of the metabolic aspects of diabetes are described in this chapter. A clear understanding of these processes is helpful for diabetes educators in order to

A Provide in-depth information to patients about diabetes, the symptoms, and metabolic effects

B Understand the actions of the nonpharmacologic and pharmacologic therapies for diabetes in order to provide both information and clinically appropriate care

C Better understand the interactions between food, activity, medications, and blood glucose levels for decision-making and to prepare persons with diabetes for self-management

D Understand the pathogenesis of the complications of diabetes and teach individuals about modifiable risk factors and symptom recognition for early treatment

4 Although hyperglycemia plays a major and preventable role in the complications of diabetes (abnormalities in the structure and function of blood vessels and nerves), other pathological processes and additional risk factors are major, and sometimes independent, etiologies (see Chapter 3, Chronic Complications of Diabetes, in Diabetes and Complications, for more information).

5 The reader is encouraged to consider the pathophysiology of diabetes not as a discrete problem of carbohydrate-insulin abnormality, but as a dynamic interplay of etiologies.

Objectives

Upon completion of this chapter, the learner will be able to

1 Describe fuel metabolism and its hormonal control.

2 Identify the groups at risk for diabetes.

3 State the diagnostic criteria for diabetes mellitus.

4 Identify the differences among the various forms of diabetes mellitus.

5 Explain the stages of development of type 1 diabetes and the implications for early intervention and prevention.

6 Explain the mechanisms by which type 2 diabetes occurs, the risk factors for its development, and mechanisms for potential prevention.

Key Definitions

1 *Adipocyte.* A fat cell that serves as the primary storage for excess calories.

2 *Genotype.* The specific description of a defined region of a chromosome.

3 *Glucagon.* A hormone produced by the alpha cells of the pancreatic islets of Langerhans and a counterregulatory hormone to insulin. Glucagon release results in an increase in the circulating glucose level by stimulating gluconeogenesis.

4 *Gluconeogenesis.* The process of glucose production in the liver from precursors such as lactate and amino acids.

5 *Glycogen.* A complex carbohydrate that serves as the primary storage form of glucose in the liver and muscle.

6 *Glycogenolysis.* The metabolic conversion of glycogen into glucose.

7 *Lactate.* An incomplete breakdown product in the anaerobic metabolism of glucose; can serve as a precursor for subsequent glucose synthesis in the process of gluconeogenesis.

8 *Substrate.* A material that may be acted upon by enzymes in a metabolic process (ie, lactate is a substrate for gluconeogenesis).

Normal Fuel Metabolism

1 Five phases of fuel homeostasis have been described by Chipkin et al.[1]

　A Phase I is the fed state (0 to 3.9 hours after meal/food consumption), in which blood glucose predominantly originates from an exogenous source.

　　• The brain and other organs use some of the glucose that has been absorbed from the gastrointestinal tract.

　　• The remaining glucose is added to hepatic, muscle, adipose, and other tissue reservoirs.

　　• Plasma insulin levels are high, glucagon levels are low, and triglyceride is synthesized in liver and adipose tissue. Insulin inhibits breakdown of glycogen and triglyceride reservoirs.

　B Phase II is the postabsorptive state (4 to 15.9 hours after food consumption), in which blood glucose originates from glycogen breakdown and hepatic gluconeogenesis.

　　• Plasma insulin levels decrease and glucagon levels increase.

　　• Energy storage ends in this phase and energy production begins.

　　• Carbohydrate and lipid stores are mobilized. Hepatic glycogen breakdown provides glucose to the brain and other tissues. Blood glucose levels are maintained.

　　• Adipocyte triglyceride begins to break down and free fatty acids (FFA) are released into the circulation and utilized by the liver and skeletal muscle as a primary energy source.

　　• The brain continues to use glucose, provided mainly by gluconeogenesis (35% to 60%) because of its inability to use FFA as fuel.

C Phase III is the early starvation state (16 to 47.9 hours after food consumption), in which blood glucose originates from hepatic gluconeogenesis and glycogenolysis.
  • Gluconeogenesis continues to produce most of the hepatic glucose.
  • In this phase of starvation, lactate makes up half of the gluconeogenetic substrate.
  • Amino acids, specifically alanine, and glycerol are other major substrates.
  • Insulin secretion is markedly suppressed and counterregulatory hormone (eg, glucagon, cortisol, growth hormone, and epinephrine) secretion is stimulated.

D Phase IV is the preliminary prolonged starvation state (48 hours to 23.9 days after food consumption), in which blood glucose originates from hepatic and renal gluconeogenesis.
  • By 60 hours of starvation, gluconeogenesis provides more than 97% of hepatic glucose output. The need for gluconeogenesis is limited in order to conserve body protein by increased reliance of muscle and other tissues on FFA and ketone bodies and a change from glucose to ketone bodies as fuel for the brain.
  • Insulin secretion is markedly suppressed and counterregulatory hormone (eg, glucagon, cortisol, growth hormone, and epinephrine) secretion is stimulated.

E Phase V is the secondary prolonged starvation state (24 to 40 days after food consumption), in which blood glucose originates from hepatic and renal gluconeogenesis, the same source as in Phase IV. In Phase V, the rate of glucose being used by the brain diminishes as does the rate of hepatic gluconeogenesis.

Definition of Diabetes Mellitus

1 *Diabetes mellitus* consists of a group of metabolic diseases characterized by inappropriate hyperglycemia resulting from defects in insulin secretion, insulin action, or both.

2 The pathogenic processes in the development of diabetes involve beta cell dysfunction, which leads to impaired insulin synthesis and/or release, and peripheral insulin resistance. The beta cell dysfunction may be due to immune-mediated insulitis, genetically determined beta cell dysfunction, or acquired beta cell dysfunction (including glucose toxicity).

3 Insulin resistance is manifested by persistent hepatic glucose production and diminished peripheral glucose disposal. Abnormal insulin signalling occurs distal to its binding to the insulin receptor with observed defects in glucokinase activity and glucose transporter translocation being noted.

4 Symptoms of acute hyperglycemia include polyuria, polydipsia, polyphagia, weight loss, blurred vision, fatigue, headache, occasional muscle cramps, and poor wound healing.

5 Signs and symptoms of chronic hyperglycemia include growth impairment; susceptibility to certain infections; and renal, retinal, peripheral vascular, connective tissue, and neuropathic syndromes.

6 Acute life-threatening consequences of diabetes include hyperglycemia with ketoacidosis (DKA), hyperosmolar hyperglycemic state (HHS), and therapy-induced hypoglycemia.

Diagnostic Criteria for Diabetes Mellitus and Other Categories of Impaired Glucose Homeostasis

1 In 1997, the Expert Committee on the Diagnosis and Classification of Diabetes Mellitus[2] updated the classification and diagnostic criteria for diabetes. Diabetes mellitus is diagnosed using any 1 of the 3 following methods and must be confirmed on a subsequent day.

   A Acute symptoms of diabetes plus casual plasma glucose concentration ≥200 mg/dL (11.1 mmol/L).
- Casual implies any time of day without regard to time since last meal.
- The classic symptoms of diabetes include polyuria, polydipsia, polyphagia, and unexplained weight loss.

   B Fasting plasma glucose ≥126 mg/dL (7.0 mmol/L). Fasting is defined as no caloric intake for at least 8 hours.

   C Two-hour plasma glucose ≥200mg/dL (11.1 mmol/L) during a 75-g oral glucose tolerance test (OGTT).

2 Impaired Fasting Glucose (IFG) is diagnosed when fasting glucose levels are ≥110 mg/dL (6.1 mmol/L) but <126 mg/dL (7.0 mmol/L). IFG represents a metabolic stage of impaired glucose homeostasis intermediate between normal and diabetes mellitus. IFG is not a category of diabetes mellitus.

3 Impaired Glucose Tolerance (IGT) is diagnosed when 2-hour OGTT values are ≥140 mg/dL (7.0 mmol/L) but <200 mg/dL (11.1 mmol/L). IGT represents a metabolic stage of impaired glucose homeostasis intermediate between normal and diabetes mellitus. IGT is not a category of diabetes mellitus, but is associated with increased macrovascular disease.

4 The 1997 classifications focus on the etiology of this heterogeneous disease rather than the treatment. The terminology has been revised in the following ways:

   A The terms insulin-dependent diabetes mellitus (IDDM) and noninsulin-dependent diabetes mellitus (NIDDM) are eliminated.

   B Arabic numerals and lowercase letters replace the Roman numerals and capital "T"; thus, Type I diabetes becomes type 1 diabetes, and Type II diabetes becomes type 2 diabetes.

Classification of Diabetes Mellitus

1 The following characteristics define *type 1 diabetes*:

   A Develops at any age, but most cases are diagnosed before the age of 30 years.

   B Characterized by autoimmune destruction of the beta cells of the islets of Langerhans with resulting absolute insulin deficiency.

   C Dependent on exogenous insulin to prevent ketoacidosis and sustain life.

   D Affected individuals experience significant weight loss, polyuria, and polydipsia characterized by the abrupt signs and symptoms associated with marked hyperglycemia and the strong propensity for the development of ketoacidosis.

   E Coma and death can result from a delayed diagnosis and/or treatment.

2 The following characteristics define type 2 diabetes:

   A Approximately 90% of patients in the US with diabetes have type 2 diabetes, with disproportionate representation among the elderly and certain ethnic populations.

   B Usually diagnosed after the age of 30 years, but can occur at any age. Onset in adolescents is becoming more common among individuals in the Hispanic and African American communities. Type 2 diabetes now accounts for 30% to 50% of childhood-onset diabetes.

   C Frequently asymptomatic at the time of diagnosis, but as many as 20% may present with end-organ complications (eg, retinopathy, neuropathy, and nephropathy).

   D Endogenous insulin levels may be normal, increased, or decreased; the need for exogenous insulin is variable.

   E Insulin resistance is typically present with impaired glucose tolerance in the initial stages.

   F Not prone to ketosis except in rare cases of severe physiologic stress.

   G Approximately 50% of men and 70% of women are obese at the time of diagnosis.[3]

3 Other type of diabetes are

   A *Secondary diabetes* is diagnosed when diabetes occurs as a result of other disorders or treatments. Treatment of these other disorders or discontinuation of diabetogenic agents may result in amelioration of the diabetes. However, frequently it is impossible to reverse the underlying disorder or stop the offending agent, in which case the therapy is similar to diabetes therapy in general using the modalities of medical nutrition therapy, exercise, and medications. The following disorders are classified as secondary diabetes:

      • Known genetic defects associated with Maturity-Onset Diabetes of the Young (MODY), glycogen synthase deficiency, and mitochondrial DNA markers.

      • Pancreatic disorders such as hemochromatosis, chronic pancreatitis, and pancreatectomy.

      • Hormonal disorders such as Cushing syndrome (excess amounts of corticosteroids), pheochromocytoma (excess catecholamines), and acromegaly (excess growth hormone).

      • Other disorders such as cystic fibrosis, congenital rubella syndrome, and Down syndrome.

      • Concomitant diabetogenic drug therapy (eg, glucocorticoids, pentamidine).

   B *Gestational diabetes* is a diagnosis of diabetes mellitus that applies only to women in whom glucose intolerance develops or is first discovered during pregnancy.

      • After pregnancy, the diagnostic classification may be changed to previous abnormality of glucose tolerance, type 1 or type 2 diabetes or impaired glucose tolerance.

      • Women whose diabetes predated the pregnancy should not be included in the gestational diabetes classification.

      • The occurrence of gestational diabetes increases the future risk for progression to type 2 diabetes, or, rarely, type 1 diabetes.

Natural History and Pathophysiology of Type 1 Diabetes

1 Type 1 diabetes results from an autoimmune attack on the beta cell.[4]

    A Type 1 diabetes is characterized by the abrupt onset of clinical signs and symptoms associated with marked hyperglycemia and the strong propensity for the development of ketoacidosis.

    B The disease begins to develop long before the clinical signs become evident.

2 Pathologic and biochemical changes may occur as long as 9 years before the clinical onset of type 1 diabetes. The 5 stages of development are shown in Table 1.1.

Table 1.1. Pathophysiologic Stages in the Development of Type 1 Diabetes

Stage 1	Genetic predisposition
Stage 2	Environmental trigger
Stage 3	Active autoimmunity
Stage 4	Progressive beta cell dysfunction
Stage 5	Overt diabetes mellitus

    A There is a genetic propensity for type 1 diabetes.

- The risk of type 1 diabetes in the general population ranges from 1 in 400 to 1 in 1000.[5] That risk is substantially increased (from approximately 1 in 20 to 1 in 50) in the offspring of individuals with diabetes.
- The genetic predisposition to type 1 diabetes is the result of the combination of HLA-DQ coded genes for disease susceptibility offset by genes that are related to disease resistance. Genes that produce resistance are frequently dominant over those that produce disease susceptibility.
- HLA-DR3 and/or HLA-DR4 appear to be present in greater than 90% of Caucasians with type 1 diabetes. However, 95% of these individuals are found to have HLA-DQA1*0301, HLA-DQA1*0302. This HLA genotype is strongly associated with the occurrence of type 1 diabetes among African American, Caucasian, and Japanese populations.
- Dominant protection from developing diabetes results from the presence of the genotype HLA-DQ B-1*0602 or HLA-DQW1.2.
- Not all individuals at genetic risk for type 1 diabetes ultimately develop the disease.
- Although 40% of Caucasian individuals express the DR-3 or DR-4 haplotype, fewer than 1% ultimately develop diabetes.[4]
- A 50% discordance rate of type 1 diabetes exists between identical twins, suggesting that specific genes are necessary but not sufficient conditions for its development.

B A trigger is necessary for the expression of the genetic propensity for type 1 diabetes; environmental triggers have long been suspected.

- Viral triggers are suggested by the association of type 1 diabetes with congenital rubella syndrome and Coxsackie B4 infection.
- Bovine serum albumin (BSA) is thought to be an environmental trigger by many investigators.
- BSA-specific antibodies are found in the majority of children with newly diagnosed diabetes. Thus, early exposure to cow's milk may be a potential determinant of subsequent type 1 diabetes, increasing disease risk by as much as 1.5 times.[6] (See Chapter 5, Lifestyle for Diabetes Prevention, in Diabetes in the Life Cycle and Research, for more information on this topic.)
- Structural similarities exist between BSA and an islet cell surface antigen referred to as ICA-69. The cross-reactivity of circulating anti-BSA antibodies with ICA-69 would provide a link between the environmental trigger and the subsequent development of autoimmunity, causing type 1 diabetes.
- Additional environmental factors that have been suggested as triggers for type 1 diabetes include sex steroids as seen in puberty and during pregnancy, environmental toxins (including N-nitroso derivatives and the rodenticide vacor), or possibly insulin itself.[7]

C Regardless of the trigger, early type 1 diabetes is first identified by the appearance of active autoimmunity directed against pancreatic beta cells and their products.

- Fifty percent of relatives with high titer islet cell antibodies (ICAs) have diabetes within 5 years of follow up. ICA negativity has a 99.9% probability of freedom from the development of type 1 diabetes.
- *ICAs* are composed of a variety of specific islet cell antibodies that may interact with diabetic serum. Many measurements of titers are currently available from commercial laboratories.
- *Glutamic acid decarboxylase* (GAD), a $64\,000\ M_r$ protein appears to be the best immunologic predictor for the future development of type 1 diabetes.[8]
- Additional islet cell autoantibodies that may play a permissive or pathologic role in the causation of type 1 diabetes are shown in Table 1.2.
- There is also an immunologic attack on insulin, the product of the beta cell.
- Seventy-eight percent of future cases of type 1 diabetes found in ICA-positive individuals arose from the subset with multiple autoantibodies; thus, the combination of positive antibody titers provides both increased sensitivity and specificity for disease progression.[9]

D The combination of autoimmune attack on beta cells and on insulin by insulin autoantibodies (IAAs) progressively diminishes the effective circulating insulin level.

- Before the clinical onset of diabetes mellitus, intravenous (IV) glucose tolerance testing demonstrates a progressive decline in first-phase insulin secretion (the insulin released within the first 5 minutes following an IV glucose stimulus) in individuals with positive immunologic markers. More than 50% of individuals with positive ICAs, but normal glucose tolerance tests have first-phase insulin secretion that falls within the 10th percentile of the normal population.[10]
- Hyperglycemia and symptoms consistent with the diagnosis of diabetes mellitus develop only after >90% of the secretory capacity of the beta cell mass has been destroyed.

E The clinical onset of diabetes may be abrupt, but the pathophysiologic insult is a slow, progressive phenomenon.

- At any time during the progressive decline in beta cell function, overt diabetes may be precipitated by either acute illness or stress, thus increasing the insulin demand beyond the reserve of the damaged islet cell mass.
- *Latent autoimmune diabetes of aging* (LADA) may account for as many as 10% of cases of insulin-requiring diabetes in older individuals and represents a slowly progressive form of type 1 diabetes.

Table 1.2. Islet Cell Antibodies (ICAs) Observed in Type 1 Diabetes

Autoantigen	T-Cell Reactivity	Description
GM2-1	?	Nonspecific; in all islet cells
Glutamic acid decarboxylase (GAD)	Positive	Present as GAD-65, GAD-67, and 64 000 M_r antibodies
Insulin	Positive	Insulin autoantibodies (IAAs)
ICA-69 (IPM-1)	?	Homologous with bovine serum albumin (BSA)
38 000 M_r	Positive	Secretory granule related
52 000 M_r	?	Rubella associated
Carboxypeptidase H	?	Secretory granule related
GLUT	?	Inhibition of glucose-stimulated insulin secretion

- Hyperglycemia will ensue until such time as the acute illness or stress is resolved; then the individual may revert to a compensated state for a variable time period in which the beta cell mass is sufficient to maintain normal glycemia. This "honeymoon period" is a variable period of noninsulin dependency following acute decompensation.
- Continued beta cell destruction occurs and ultimately the individual will require insulin within 3 to 12 months, after which the person will have permanent diabetes.

F Identifying these multiple stages of development of type 1 diabetes provides a provocative framework for potential interventions that focus on prevention and cure.
- Identifying HLA markers may allow recognition of populations at risk at the time of birth.
- Developing specific vaccines against identified environmental triggers, or the simple avoidance of suspected environmental toxins such as bovine serum albumin, may prevent triggering of autoimmunity.
- Identifying active autoimmunity by measuring islet cell antibodies may serve as a marker for individuals who are destined to develop diabetes.
- The National Institutes of Health has embarked upon the *Diabetes Prevention Trial–Type 1* (DPT-1) to include screening first-degree relatives of probands with type 1 diabetes via ICA measurement, including anti-GAD, and performing IV glucose tolerance testing with measurement of first-phase insulin release.

Individuals are stratified according to risks and interventions with either oral insulin or subcutaneous insulin in an effort to prevent the ultimate development of type 1 diabetes.

Natural History and Pathophysiology of Type 2 Diabetes

1 Ascertainment of type 2 diabetes remains extremely poor, with almost 30% of those affected being undiagnosed.[11] Microvascular complications are found in approximately 20% of newly diagnosed individuals with type 2 diabetes.

   A Type 2 diabetes may be present, on average, for about 6.5 years prior to its clinical identification and treatment.[12]

   B The prevalence of coronary artery disease in those with type 2 diabetes is twice that of the nondiabetic population, and cardiovascular and total mortality are 2- to 3-fold greater than in nondiabetic individuals.

2 Heredity plays a major role in the expression of type 2 diabetes.

   A Although there is no recognized HLA linkage, offspring of individuals with type 2 diabetes have a 15% chance of developing the disease and a 30% risk of developing impaired glucose tolerance.[5]

   B A greater than 90% concordance rate exists between monozygotic twins if one has type 2 diabetes, suggesting the primacy of the genetic defect in this form of the disease.

3 Identification of specific gene defects in certain groups with exceptionally high prevalence of type 2 diabetes has resulted in their designation as secondary forms of diabetes.

   A The Pima Indians have a 50% prevalence of type 2 diabetes, with insulin resistance and hyperinsulinemia inherited as an autosomal trait.[13]

   B *Maturity-Onset Diabetes of the Young (MODY)* is a series of 5 familial disorders characterized by early onset and mild hyperglycemia. Three specific genetic defects have been identified on chromosomes 7, 12, and 20.[14]

4 *Type 2 diabetes* is a heterogeneous disorder characterized by variable plasma insulin levels with associated hyperglycemia and peripheral insulin resistance. This disorder has been described as the metabolic syndrome or the insulin resistance syndrome and includes numerous factors associated with increased cardiovascular risk (see Chapter 6, Macrovascular Disease, in Diabetes and Complications).

5 Type 2 diabetes may be divided into several specific defects:

   A Primary beta cell dysfunction resulting in insulin deficiency (inadequate insulin to control blood glucose levels)

   B Insulin receptor abnormalities (rare)

   C Specific postreceptor defects, including altered glucose transporter function and specific enzymatic defects that modulate intracellular insulin activity, resulting in insulin resistance.

6 Limitation in beta cell response to hyperglycemia appears to be the cornerstone of the pathophysiology of type 2 diabetes.[15]

A A 50% reduction in beta cell mass is seen in individuals with type 2 diabetes compared with controls, particularly when the degree of obesity is also taken into account. No evidence of autoimmune insulitis is found within these beta cells, but the expected degree of hypertrophy and hyperfunction caused by chronic hyperglycemia is distinctly absent.

B Abnormal beta cell recognition of glucose and its subsequent linkage to insulin synthesis and secretion are specific mechanisms by which the beta cell plays a critical role in type 2 diabetes.

C Intrinsic abnormalities in patterns of insulin secretion are noted in most individuals with type 2 diabetes. The packaging and secretion of insulin appear to be progressive abnormalities in the transition from normal to impaired glucose tolerance and subsequently to type 2 diabetes.

D Abnormal secretion of the insulin precursor, *proinsulin,* has been noted in multiple populations.

E Acquired defects in beta cell activity have been noted in response to hyperglycemia and referred to as *glucose toxicity.*
  - Beta cells chronically exposed to hyperglycemia and to increased free fatty acids become progressively less efficient in responding to subsequent glucose challenges.[16]
  - Thus, beta cell dysfunction may be either primary or acquired in the pathogenesis of type 2 diabetes; however, it remains a necessary component of carbohydrate intolerance in any event.

7 A second essential trait of type 2 diabetes is the presence of resistance to the biologic activity of insulin noted in both liver and peripheral tissues.[17] Severe insulin resistance exists years before the onset of hyperglycemia.

A Resistance to the biologic activity of insulin may result in hyperglycemia with progressively increasing requirements for insulin secretion resulting in expression of either glucose toxicity or some genetic limitation in beta cell activity.

B The relative roles of insulin resistance and insulin deficiency remain highly controversial and are frequently presented in the literature.[18]

8 In the fasting state, circulating blood glucose is maintained by hepatic glucose production via glycogenolysis and gluconeogenesis. Insulin suppresses these processes in a marked dose-response fashion.

A Those with type 2 diabetes have a substantial shift to the right of the dose-response curves, with a decrease in both the sensitivity and response of the system.

B Thus, regardless of circulating insulin levels, type 2 diabetes is associated with a persistent hepatic glucose production that increases fasting and post-absorptive glucose levels.

9 Studies[15] using a euglycemic hyperinsulinemic clamp show both decreased sensitivity and response in peripheral glucose disposal in individuals with type 2 diabetes compared with nondiabetic controls.

10 Early suggestions of impaired insulin receptor function have not been demonstrated. Rare individuals have been identified as having altered insulin receptor structure or function. However, in the vast majority of individuals with type 2 diabetes, insulin binding to its receptor, insulin receptor number, and insulin receptor activity appear to be entirely normal.[17]

11 These premises, along with the public health demands of recognizing an insidious disorder associated with substantial morbidity and mortality, have led the National Institutes of Health to propose a prevention trial for type 2 diabetes.[19]

A *The Diabetes Prevention Program* (DPP) screened over 14,000 high-risk individuals for the presence of impaired glucose tolerance.

B Subsequent interventions with intensive lifestyle modifications (eating habits, exercise, and subsequent weight loss) versus a pharmacologic intervention (metformin) to improve endogenous insulin action are aimed at ameliorating the specific defects prior to decompensation to a hyperglycemic state. Results are expected to be available by the end of 2002.

Key Educational Considerations

1 *Diabetes mellitus* is a syndrome of altered fuel metabolism characterized by inappropriate hyperglycemia resulting from defects in insulin secretion, insulin action, or both, and associated with chronic microvascular and macrovascular complications.

2 Newly revised diagnostic criteria and classification of disease have been adopted.

3 *Type 1 diabetes* is an autoimmune disorder resulting in destruction of pancreatic beta cells, requiring insulin therapy to prevent ketoacidosis and death.

4 *Type 2 diabetes* is a heterogeneous disorder in which specific secondary genetic causes of the metabolic syndrome are being rapidly identified.

5 Type 2 diabetes is characterized by variable beta cell function (insulin deficiency) and peripheral insulin resistance.

Self-Review Questions

1 Describe normal metabolism in each of the 5 phases of full homeostasis.
2 Define diabetes mellitus based on the 3 methods used in its diagnosis.
3 Describe 3 differences between type 1 diabetes and type 2 diabetes.
4 Describe the natural history of type 1 diabetes and type 2 diabetes.

References

1 Chipkin SR, Kelly KL, Ruderman NB. Hormone-fuel interrelationships: fed state, starvation, and diabetes mellitus. In: Kahn CR, Weir GS, eds. Joslin's Diabetes Mellitus. 13th ed. Philadelphia: Lea & Febiger; 1994:97-115.

2 Expert Committee on the Diagnosis and Classification of Diabetes Mellitus. Report of the expert committee on the diagnosis and classification of diabetes mellitus. Diabetes Care. 2001; 24(suppl 1):S5-S20.

3 Harris MI. Classification, diagnostic criteria, and screening for diabetes. In: National Diabetes Data Group. Diabetes in American. 2nd ed. Bethesda, Md: National Institutes of Health, National Institute of Diabetes and Digestive and Kidney Disorder; 1995. NIH publication 95-1468:16.

4 Thai A-C, Eisenbarth GS. Natural history of IDDM. Diabetes Rev. 1993;1:1-14.

5 Redondo MJ, Fain PR, Eisenbarth GS. Genetics of type 1A diabetes. Recent Prog Horm Res. 2001;56:69-89.

6 Wasnuth HE, Kolb H. Cow's milk and immune-mediated diabetes. Proc Nutr Soc. 2000;59:573-579.

7 Vaarala O, Hyoty H, Akerblom HK. Environmental factors in the aetiology of childhood diabetes. Diabetes Nutr Metab. 1999;12(2):75-85.

8 Atkinson MA, MacLaren NK, Scharp DW, Lacy PE, Riley WJ. 64,000 Mr autoantibodies as predictors of insulin-dependent diabetes. Lancet. 1990;35:1357-1360.

9 Bingley PJ, Christie MR, Bonifacio E, et al. Combined analysis of autoantibodies improves prediction of IDDM in islet antibody positive relatives. Diabetes. 1994;43:1304-1310.

10 Maclaren NK. How, when and why to predict IDDM. Diabetes. 1988;37:1591-1594.

11 Centers for Disease Control and Prevention. National diabetes fact sheet. US Department of Health and Human Services, Centers for Disease Control and Prevention, Division of Diabetes Translation. Atlanta;1997.

12 Matthews DR. The natural history of diabetes-related complications: the UKPDS experience. Diabetes Obes Metab. 1999;1(suppl 2):S7-S13.

13 Tripathy D, Carlsson AL, Lehto M, Isomaa B, Tuomi T, Groop L. Insulin secretion and insulin sensitivity in diabetic subgroups: studies in the prediabetic and diabetic state. Diabetologia. 2000;43:1476-1483.

14 Froguel P, Velho G. Genetic determinants of type 2 diabetes. Recent Prog Horm Res. 2001;56:91-105.

15 Weir GC, Laybutt DR, Kaneto H, et al. Beta-cell adaptation and decompensation during the progression of diabetes. Diabetes. 2001;50(suppl 1):S154-S159.

16 Saltiel AR. New perspectives into the molecular pathogenesis and treatment of type 2 diabetes. Cell. 2001;104:517-529.

17 Gerich JE. Is insulin resistance the principal cause of type 2 diabetes? Diabetes Obes Metab. 1999;1:257-263.

18 Taylor SI, Accili D, Imai Y. Insulin resistance or insulin deficiency. Which is the primary cause of NIDDM? Diabetes. 1994;43:735-740.

19 The Diabetes Prevention Program Research Group. The Diabetes Prevention Program. Baseline characteristics of the randomized cohort. Diabetes Care. 2000;23:1619-1629.

Suggested Readings

Flier JS. Diabetes. The missing link with obesity? Nature. 2001;409:292-293.

Fujimoto WY, Bergstrom RW, Boyko EJ, et al. Preventing diabetes-applying pathophysiological and epidemiological evidence. Br J Nutr. 2000;84(suppl 2):173-176.

Ong KK, Dunger DB. Thrifty genotypes and phenotypes in the pathogenesis of type 2 diabetes. J Pediatr Endocrinol Metab. 2000;13(suppl 6):1419-1424.

Learning Assessment: Post-Test Questions

Pathophysiology of the Diabetes Disease State   **1**

1 Gluconeogenesis is the:
   A Mechanism of breaking down complex carbohydrate for storage
   B Process of glucose production in the liver from precursors
   C Attachment of insulin with glucose at cell receptor sites
   D Transport of glucose across cell membrane for cell usage

2 Glycogenolysis is the metabolic conversion of:
   A Glycogen into glucose
   B Glucagon into glucose
   C Glucose into glycogen
   D Glucose into glucagon

3 A characteristic of the normal Phase II postabsorbtive state is:
   A Plasma insulin levels are high and glucagon levels are low
   B Triglyceride and free fatty acids are stored in the adipocyte
   C Carbohydrate and lipid stores are mobilized
   D Renal gluconeogenesis contributes to high blood glucose levels

4 Which of the following individuals would be diagnosed with diabetes mellitus using the present criteria on a subsequent day:
   A A 44-year-old woman with unexplained weight loss, fatigue, and casual plasma glucose concentrations of 180 mg/dL and 170 mg/dL
   B A 50-year-old asymptomatic male with a fasting plasma glucose of 138 mg/dL and 146 mg/dL
   C A 28-year-old male with a 2-hour plasma glucose (OGTT) of 160 mg/dL and 140 mg/dL
   D A 60-year-old female with casual plasma glucose concentrations of 145 mg/ dL and 130 mg/dL

5 Which statement best describes the differences in the characteristics between type 1 and type 2 diabetes:
   A Persons with type 2 diabetes usually require lower doses of insulin because of the presence of some functioning beta cells
   B Persons with type 1 diabetes may be asymptomatic at the time of diagnosis but rapidly develop complications
   C Persons with type 1 diabetes require endogenous insulin, and persons with type 2 diabetes utilize exogenous insulin to regulate blood glucose levels
   D Autoimmune factors are more likely to be a cause or contributing factor for type 1 diabetes than for type 2 diabetes

6 JJ, a 16-year-old male, is frequently leaving class, going to the bathroom to urinate, and stopping by the water fountain for a drink. Despite the fact that he eats a lot in school and at home, he is losing weight. JJ is exhibiting symptoms of:
   A Hyperglycemia
   B Hypoglycemia
   C Ketoacidosis
   D Hyperosmolarity

7 People who do not have diabetes can have impaired fasting blood glucose values. One example of this is:
   A A school-aged child with FBSs of 86 and 89 mg/dL
   B An active teenager with FBSs of 101 and 103 mg/dL
   C An employed adult with FBSs of 122 and 125 mg/dL
   D An elderly adult with FBSs of 140 and 142 mg/dL

8 The pathophysiological states in the stages of development of type 1 diabetes include all of the following except:
  A Peripheral insulin resistance
  B An environmental trigger
  C A genetic predisposition
  D Beta cell immune attack

9 Beta cell function in persons with type 2 diabetes is best characterized by:
  A Hypertrophy and hyperfunction caused by hyperglycemia
  B 10% to 20% reduction in cell mass leading to diminished response to hyperglycemia
  C Altered or impaired insulin receptor function
  D Abnormal insulin secretion in response to impaired recognition of glucose

10 DP only eats once a day. After 16 to 24 hours her circulating blood glucose levels are maintained by production from all of the following substances, except:
  A Lactate
  B Amino acids
  C Fatty acids
  D Glycogen

11 Which of the following individuals is at greatest risk for developing type 1 diabetes?
  A A person who is shown to have a genetic predisposition for type 1 diabetes
  B An identical twin in whom type 1 diabetes has developed in the other twin
  C Individuals with high levels of glutamic acid decarboxylase antibodies
  D Persons exposed to an environmental trigger independent of autoimmune factors

See next page for answer key.

Post-Test Answer Key

Pathophysiology of the Diabetes Disease State   1

1	B		**6**	A
2	A		**7**	C
3	C		**8**	A
4	B		**9**	D
5	D		**10**	D
			11	C

A Core Curriculum for Diabetes Education
Diabetes and Complications

Hyperglycemia

A Core Curriculum for Diabetes Education
Diabetes and Complications

Hyperglycemia 2

Mayer B. Davidson, MD
Charles R. Drew University
Los Angeles, California

Stephanie Schwartz, MPH, RN, CDE
Children With Diabetes .Com
Ann Arbor, Michigan

Introduction

1 Prolonged hyperglycemia can lead to two types of acute metabolic crises: *diabetic ketoacidosis* (DKA) and *hyperosmolar hyperglycemic state* (HHS). Either of these life-threatening conditions may result in an altered mental state, loss of consciousness, or possibly death. Prompt medical attention is necessary to avoid adverse outcomes. The mortality rate in patients with DKA is <5% in experienced centers, whereas the mortality rate of patients with HHS is ~15%.[1]

2 DKA is a complication that results from an absolute or relative deficiency in insulin. Occurring most frequently in persons with type 1 diabetes, DKA can occur in persons with type 2 patients as well.[2] DKA is characterized by hyperglycemia, ketosis, acidosis, and dehydration.

3 HHS is a life-threatening emergency with a high mortality rate.[3] This metabolic crisis is usually seen in the elderly or undiagnosed person with type 2 diabetes and is characterized by four main clinical features:

A Severe hyperglycemia (blood glucose >600 mg/dL [33.3 mmol/L])[1]

B Absence of ketoacidosis

C Profound dehydration

D Neurologic signs ranging from depressed sensorium to frank coma

4 Despite improved monitoring and treatments, DKA and HHS still remain significant problems. Prevention through patient education, early recognition of symptoms, and prompt efficacious treatment must be emphasized.

Objectives

Upon completion of this chapter, the learner will be able to

1 Identify the precipitating factors in DKA.

2 Describe the pathophysiology of DKA.

3 State presenting signs and symptoms of DKA.

4 Describe possible variations in initial laboratory values.

5 State 3 goals in the treatment of DKA.

6 Identify precipitating factors in HHS.

7 Describe the pathophysiology of HHS.

8 State presenting signs and symptoms of HHS.

9 State the major or primary component of treatment for HHS.

10 Explain the major differences between laboratory values found in DKA and HHS.

Diabetic Ketoacidosis

1 The characteristics of diabetic ketoacidosis (DKA) are hyperglycemia, ketosis, dehydration, and electrolyte imbalance.

2 Precipitating factors of DKA vary from individual to individual.

A Infection and illness are the precipitating factors in approximately 30% to 40% of cases.[4] Infection and illness increase production of glucocorticoids by the adrenal gland, promoting *gluconeogenesis* (production of new glucose by the liver).

Epinephrine and norepinephrine levels are also increased, which in turn cause an increase in *glycogenolysis* (breakdown of glycogen into glucose).

B Newly onset type 1 diabetes or discontinuation of or inadequate insulin dosage (either provider- or patient-directed) commonly lead to the development of DKA.
- The initial manifestation of type 1 diabetes may be DKA.
- Patients with gastrointestinal (GI) symptoms often decrease or omit their insulin doses in the mistaken belief that less insulin is needed when food intake is decreased. Because GI signs and symptoms are prominent features of DKA, decreasing insulin dosages can be dangerous.
- Insulin doses may be omitted because of fear of weight gain with improved metabolic control, attempts to lose weight, fear of hypoglycemia, or rebellion from authority.[1]
- Emotional stress may be a precipitating factor, particularly among adolescents. Neglect or mismanagement may be a deliberate call for help.
- Psychological problems complicated by eating disorders may be a factor in 20% of recurrent ketoacidosis.[1]

Pathophysiology of DKA

1 DKA is caused by profound insulin deficiency. Although small amounts of insulin may be circulating, the presence of large amounts of stress hormones (glucagon, catecholamines [eg, epinephrine and norepinephrine], cortisol, and growth hormone) render the insulin less effective. Carbohydrate, protein, and fat metabolism are all markedly affected (Figure 2.1).

A After eating, insulin deficiency impairs glucose uptake in the peripheral tissues (mainly muscle) and liver, leading to hyperglycemia. During fasting, insulin deficiency results in excess hepatic glucose production that can also lead to hyperglycemia.

B Insulin deficiency causes impaired protein synthesis and excessive protein degradation.
- The resulting increase in the gluconeogenic amino acids leads to increased hepatic glucose production (by means of gluconeogenesis) and finally hyperglycemia.
- The failure to build new protein and the increased breakdown of already formed protein are the reasons for the loss of lean body mass in uncontrolled diabetes.

C Severe insulin deficiency and increased counterregulatory hormones cause excessive hydrolysis of *triglycerides*, the stored form of fat, releasing increased amounts of free fatty acids (FFA) and glycerol. This metabolic pathway is called *lipolysis*.
- Glycerol is an important gluconeogenic precursor that leads to increasing hepatic glucose production and further hyperglycemia.
- Excessive amounts of ketone bodies (ß-hydroxybutyric acid and acetoacetic acid) are formed in the liver from the FFA with resulting ketonemia and metabolic acidosis.
- Low levels of insulin permit ketogenesis, not only by providing more FFA but also by enhancing certain critical hepatic enzymes that change FFA into ketone bodies.

Figure 2.1. Diabetic Ketoacidosis — Hyperosmolar Hyperglycemia State Pathways

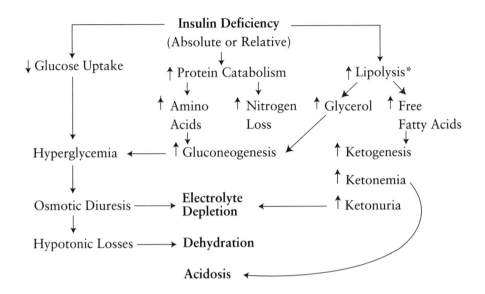

*not increased in HHS

Source: Adapted with permission from Davidson.[5]

2 Hyperglycemia leads to an osmotic diuresis, which causes hypotonic fluid losses and dehydration as well as electrolyte depletion.

   A Ketone bodies are weak acids that can be used by most tissues only to a limited extent. When this capacity is exceeded, the ketone bodies must be neutralized (buffered). As ketones continue to accumulate, the buffering capacity of the body is exhausted and acidosis supervenes.

   B The excretion of ketone bodies in the urine, a process called *ketonuria*, leads to more electrolyte depletion because cations must be eliminated along with the anionic ketone bodies to maintain electrical neutrality.

   C Twelve to 24 hours of insulin deficiency in patients with type 1 diabetes (depending on the hyperglycemic state) causes profound fluid and electrolyte losses.

      • Fluids, sodium, potassium, and chloride must be vigorously replaced in the initial hours of treatment.

      • There is controversy concerning the need for magnesium and phosphate replacement.[5]

Signs and Symptoms of Hyperglycemia

1 The symptoms of hyperglycemia may mimic other diseases or conditions. Although the symptoms of poorly controlled diabetes may be present for several days, the metabolic alterations typical of ketoacidosis usually occur within a short time frame (typically <24 hours). Occasionally, DKA may develop more acutely with no prior signs or symptoms.[1]

A Manifestations of hyperglycemia are polyuria; polydipsia; blurred vision; polyphagia, if insulin deficiency is present long enough (days to weeks); and weight loss.

B Nonspecific symptoms include weakness, lethargy, malaise, and headache.

C Gastrointestinal symptoms are nausea, vomiting, and abdominal pain. The cause of these symptoms is unclear, but they are probably related to the ketosis and/or acidotic state.

D Respiratory symptoms may include an inability to "catch one's breath" and a very deep, sometimes rapid, breathing unrelated to exertion termed *Kussmaul respirations*. This hyperventilation produces a respiratory alkalosis in a partial, but not completely successful, attempt to correct the metabolic acidosis by blowing off carbon dioxide.

2 There are no specific signs of DKA; rather, a constellation of evidence should suggest the possibility of DKA.

A Hypothermia is often found; therefore, the presence of fever suggests associated infection.

B *Hyperpnea* (deep respirations also termed Kussmaul respirations) is present in DKA and reflects a pulmonary response to acidosis.

C Acetone breath may be present. Acetoacetate, one of the ketone bodies, is converted to *acetone,* which is excreted by the lungs. It has a fruity odor that can sometimes be detected on the breath of the patient.

D *Dehydration* (intravascular volume depletion) is a common sign.
  • Dehydration can be assessed by observing for decreased neck vein filling from below when the patient is lying absolutely flat.
  • *Orthostatic hypotension* (a fall of systolic blood pressure of 20 mm Hg after 1 minute of standing) may occur as a result of decreased intravascular volume from dehydration.
  • Poor skin turgor and "soft eyeballs" are late signs of profound dehydration in adults. Poor skin turgor is seen earlier in children.

E *Acute abdomen* is a common condition marked by tenderness to palpation, diminished bowel sounds, and some muscle guarding, especially in children. A few patients may have more severe signs (absent bowel sounds, rebound tenderness, boardlike abdomen) that suggest a surgical emergency. However, in virtually every case, these signs are due to profound DKA and disappear after treatment.

F *Mentation changes* may be present. Patients may be alert, obtunded, stuporous, or in frank coma. Mentation seems to correlate best with serum osmolality, less well with glucose concentrations, and least with pH changes.

G *Hyporeflexia,* or decreased reflexes, if not present initially, may occur if during treatment the potassium level falls below normal.

H *Hypotonia,* uncoordinated ocular movements, and fixed, dilated pupils are all late signs that suggest a poor prognosis.

Initial Laboratory Values of DKA

1 After the diagnosis of DKA is made by clinical impression and testing (a finger-stick blood glucose and blood/urine test for ketone bodies), initial laboratory tests should be obtained before therapy is begun (Table 2.1).

Table 2.1. Initial Laboratory Values for Patients Experiencing DKA

Test	Result	Remarks
Plasma glucose level	Usually >300 mg/dL (>16.7 mmol/L)	Concentration not related to severity of DKA
Ketone bodies	Positive at least in undiluted plasma	Nitroprusside test measures only acetoacetate, not ß-hydroxybutyrate
Serum bicarbonate concentration	0-15 mEq/L (0-15 mmol/L)	
Arterial pH	<7.2	
Sodium concentration	Low, normal, or high	Total body depletion
Potassium concentration	Low, normal, or high	Total body depletion; heart responsive to extracellular concentration
Phosphate level	Usually normal or slightly elevated, occasionally slightly low	Associated with phosphaturia; marked decrease in levels of both serum and urine phosphates following treatment
Creatinine, BUN* concentrations	Usually mildly increased	May be prerenal; spurious increases in creatinine level by acetoacetate in some automated methods
White blood cell count	Usually increased	Possibility of leukemoid reaction (even in absence of infection); >10% band forms usually signify severe infection
Amylase value	Often increased	Predominant form is of salivary gland origin
Hemoglobin, hematocrit, total protein values	Often increased	Secondary to contracted plasma volume
AST (SGOT),† ALT (SGPT),‡ alkaline phosphatase values	Can be elevated	Nonspecific and reversible

*BUN = blood urea nitrogen
†AST = aspartate aminotransferase (previously SGOT, serum glutamic oxaloacetic transaminase)
‡ALT = alanine aminotransferase (previously SGPT, serum glutamic pyruvic transaminase)

Source: Adapted with permission from Davidson.[5]

2 Normal values may vary in relation to the methodology of the test procedure used in an institution.

   A Glucose concentrations are usually >300 mg/dL (>16.7 mmol/L). This value is not a good index of the severity of DKA. Lower glucose levels are not uncommon, especially in children, pregnant women, and patients who have been vomiting frequently.

   B The test for ketone bodies is semiquantitative and involves the development of a purple color when serum or plasma is added to the reagent nitroprusside.

- Typically, the serum is serially diluted until a dilution is found in which no purple color is seen. The result is usually expressed as the last dilution that produces a 1+ reaction (eg, 1:8).
- Nitroprusside reacts only with acetoacetate, not with ß-hydroxybutyrate. These two ketones exist in equilibrium, with the latter in excess by three- to fivefold in DKA.
- This test for ketones can only be used to diagnose DKA; it is not useful in monitoring response to therapy because the excess ß-hydroxybutyrate is converted back to acetoacetate as the patient improves biochemically.

   C The serum bicarbonate (HCO_3) concentration will be low, usually less than 15 mEq/L, reflecting acidosis.

   D The pH is obtained on an arterial blood gas determination and will be low (less than 7.20), reflecting acidosis.

   E The carbon dioxide pressure (PCO_2) is obtained by an arterial gas determination and will be low (less than 35 mm Hg), reflecting the hyperventilatory response to the metabolic acidosis.

   F Even though loss of total body sodium (Na^+) is profound, the serum sodium level can be low, normal, or high because the sodium level depends on the amount of total body water (H_2O).

- The sodium concentration at a particular time will reflect the relative amounts of water and sodium lost and replaced up to that point.
- If the deficit of water is greater than that of sodium, the sodium level will be high; if the deficit of sodium is greater than that of water, the sodium level will be low; if the deficits are approximately equal, the sodium level will be normal.

   G The serum potassium (K^+) level can also be low, normal, or high despite a profound loss of potassium.

- The potassium level does not reflect the relative amounts of water lost but depends on the balance between the amount of potassium lost in the urine and other factors that raise the potassium level, such as the lack of insulin, which allows potassium to remain in the circulation rather than enter cells.
- If potassium entrance from the cells into the circulation exceeds excretion, serum potassium level may be high.
- Total body depletion of potassium always occurs regardless of the initial serum level.

   H Phosphate concentrations are usually high or high-normal initially, and decrease, sometimes markedly, to very low levels over the next day or two.

   I Creatinine and blood urea nitrogen (BUN) concentrations are usually mildly increased because of the dehydration and prerenal azotemia. After rehydration, elevated creatinine and BUN levels indicate the presence of renal insufficiency prior to DKA.

J Hemoglobin, hematocrit, and total protein values are often mildly elevated, reflecting the decreased plasma volume (dehydration).

K White blood cell (WBC) counts are usually increased, occasionally to very high levels. This increase does not necessarily reflect an ongoing infection, since DKA itself often causes a rise in white count. However, if a differential count is performed, >10% band forms (immature WBC) almost always denote a severe infection, whereas <10% band forms usually do not.

L Amylase values are usually increased. This increase does not reflect pancreatitis because in DKA, salivary glands, not the pancreas, release most of the amylase.

M Liver function tests often produce mildly elevated values. This elevation does not necessarily reflect acute or chronic liver damage because the values usually return to normal in several weeks (see Table 2.1).

Treatment of DKA

1 The goals of treatment of DKA are to (1) correct fluid and electrolyte disturbances, (2) provide adequate insulin to restore and maintain normal glucose metabolism and correct acidosis, (3) prevent complications resulting from the treatment of DKA, and (4) provide patient and family education and follow-up.

2 The treatment of *mild DKA* (ie, patients who can ingest and retain oral fluids without difficulty) should focus on rehydration, euglycemia, and education. If the patient or family can provide accurate blood glucose values and results of urine ketone tests, therapy provided by a knowledgeable healthcare professional over the phone may prevent a hospitalization or emergency room visit.

A Oral hydration, 3 to 5 oz per hour, is recommended if the patient is not vomiting.
   - Fluids may be given in small quantities every 20 to 30 minutes.
   - Although sugar-free fluids may be offered if the blood glucose levels are above 250 to 300 mg/dL (13.9 to 16.7 mmol/L), some programs advocate the use of sugar-containing liquids regardless of the blood glucose level. It is more important to prevent or treat the dehydration than the hyperglycemia (although the latter will maintain an osmotic diuresis that leads to continued loss of fluid if not eventually controlled).

B Patients with mild DKA require supplemental insulin. If the hyperglycemia is unaccompanied by ketosis, a proportionately smaller amount of insulin is required.
   - Insulin doses for children should be supplemented with 0.25 to 0.5 units/kg of regular insulin every 4 to 6 hours or rapid-acting insulin every 3 to 4 hours as needed.
   - The supplemental dose of insulin for adults will vary between 4 to 10 units or 10% to 20% of the usual total daily dose. The actual dose will depend on the patient's known sensitivity to insulin.

C Education regarding self-management during illness and stress management is essential to prevent DKA (see Chapter 8, Illness and Surgery, in Diabetes Management Therapies).

3 *Moderate DKA* (ie, patients who cannot retain oral fluids) and *severe DKA* (ie, patients with altered mentation) require immediate emergency treatment.

A In the rare situation in which a cardiac or respiratory arrest has occurred, the first step is to ensure an adequate airway and to assess and maintain respiratory function (and oxygen delivery). In all cases, circulation should be maintained by ensuring appropriate fluid volume replacement.[5,6]

B The diagnosis of DKA requires the presence of urine or serum ketone bodies and lowered arterial pH or serum bicarbonate level. The presence of hyperglycemia can be established by measurement of the capillary blood glucose level.

C A preliminary history and rapid physical examination (eg, vital signs, weight, blood pressure in the supine and upright positions, and pulse rate) may be obtained to confirm clinical findings and to identify other emergency measures that may be needed.

D Baseline laboratory data should be obtained without delay, including measurements of serum electrolyte values (with calculated anion gap); blood urea nitrogen/creatinine levels; serum ketones and calcium and phosphorus concentrations; arterial blood gas determination; a complete blood cell count with differential; and electrocardiogram.[1]

E After the preliminary evaluation has been made and therapy initiated, a more thorough examination needs to be performed. Precipitating causes may be identified.

4 General principles of treatment apply to almost all patients in a compromised hyperglycemic state.

A Bladder catheterization is generally not desirable. A patient who is alert will usually cooperate with voiding as required.
- If patients cannot produce urine initially, they are often successful after several hours of rehydration.
- If there is no urine flow after 4 hours of appropriate rehydration, bladder catheterization is usually warranted.
- In small infants and children, urine may be obtained through the use of urine-collection bags.

B In most patients, hypovolemia is the most acute and critical problem. The largest practical intravenous line for the rapid administration of saline must be started and its potency maintained.

C An electrocardiogram (ECG) is important, especially with leads II, V^1, or V^2. The T wave configuration aids in determining serum potassium status on admission and usually allows for earlier decisions regarding potassium therapy (Figure 2.2).
- Hypokalemia causes low or flattened T waves or U waves.
- Hyperkalemia causes peaked T waves and, if markedly elevated, a widened QRS interval.
- Serial ECG tracings will reflect changes in potassium levels as therapy proceeds. This information is available immediately before values are returned from the laboratory.
- Ongoing telemetry or placement on a telemetry unit may be warranted depending on the severity of DKA.

D Placement of a nasogastric tube should be considered in a patient who is stuporous or comatose, or who has signs of gastric dilatation, to prevent aspiration should the patient vomit.

Figure 2.2. T Wave Configuration

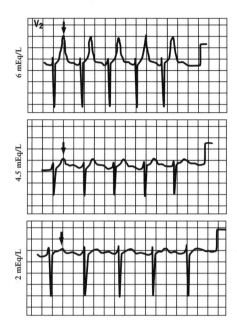

Relationship between serum concentration of potassium (K) and T wave configurations.

Source: Reproduced with permission from Davidson.[5]

E A flowsheet of pertinent lab values and actions taken is an absolute necessity to provide parameters that can be followed sequentially and in an organized fashion by different observers.

5 Fluid and electrolyte replacement is based on specific needs.

  A Adequate fluid replacement is critical for lowering glucose concentrations. Hyperglycemia will persist (even with appropriate insulin therapy) if fluid replacement is inadequate.

  B Considerations should include maintenance needs, replacement requirements, and ongoing losses.

  C Initial fluid replacement should be made with one-half normal (0.45%) or normal (0.9%) saline.

- For adults, the initial fluid replacement level depends on the degree of dehydration and cardiovascular status. In general, 1 to 2 L should be delivered in the first 1 to 2 hours and then the patient's status should be reassessed.[4-7]

- The quantities for adults are not appropriate for children. Many specialists prefer to state all values for children on the basis of kilograms of body weight. The usual calculation for fluid replacement in children is 10 to 20 mL/kg of body weight in the first hour. If no urination occurs, 20 mL/kg of body weight of fluid is given during the second and third hours as well, followed by routine fluid replacement calculated on maintenance plus deficit.

D As soon as the serum glucose level is decreased to approximately 300 mg/dL (16.7 mmol/L), intravenous fluids should be changed to contain glucose (usually D5/.45NS). Acidosis almost always persists longer than marked hyperglycemia during treatment. Therefore, adequate amounts of insulin must continue to be given (and glucose concentrations supported) until the acidosis is treated appropriately.

E Hypokalemia, if not treated properly, can lead to death.

- Potassium (K^+) should be given immediately if hypokalemia is present as determined by ECG changes or initial laboratory findings. Because of the total body potassium depletion associated with DKA, all patients with urine flow eventually need potassium repletion.

- Potassium may be added in the second to fourth hour of treatment or sooner, depending on T wave changes confirmed by laboratory values.

- Potassium replacement is based on serum potassium levels. Twenty to 40 mEq of potassium is added to a liter of fluid being infused depending on the serum potassium level. One half is sometimes given as potassium chloride and the other half as potassium phosphate. Some treatment regimens use only potassium chloride for potassium replacement, especially if the initial phosphate (PO_4) level is high or high-normal on admission, as is most often the case.

- As therapy is begun, potassium concentrations can decline rapidly from those initially obtained because of the expansion of the intravascular volume and increased renal excretion due to improved perfusion of the kidneys, both secondary to rehydration. Increased potassium entry into cells also occurs secondary to insulin administration. When the serum potassium level is <3.0 mEq/L (<3.0 mmol/L), adding more than 40 mEq (40 mmol/L) of potassium to a liter of infused fluid may be done, but the patient must be placed on a cardiac monitor.

- Patients should be carefully observed for clinically significant signs of hypokalemia including skeletal weakness progressing to paralysis, rapid diminution or absence of deep tendon reflexes, arrhythmias, and shallow, gasping respirations (in contrast to deep Kussmaul respirations).

- Continuous, frequent monitoring of ECG status and serum potassium concentration is essential to guide therapy.

F Phosphate (PO_4) levels should be measured. Some experts recommend replacing phosphate when PO_4 is low or low-normal by using potassium phosphate. Doses exceeding 1.5 mEq/L (1.5 mmol/L)/kg of body weight per 24 hours may cause hypocalcemia.

G Treatment with sodium bicarbonate ($NaHCO_3$) is controversial and is not recommended by most diabetologists.

- Some experts recommend sodium bicarbonate in severe metabolic acidosis, as indicated by an arterial pH of 7.0 or less or a serum bicarbonate level of less than 5 mEq/L (5 mmol/L). Even in this situation, a clinical benefit has not been shown with sodium bicarbonate therapy,[7] and potassium levels will drop faster and must be monitored closely. A review of the literature suggested that cerebral edema is more likely if bicarbonate is given.[8]

- Rapid infusions, or large amounts of sodium bicarbonate over a short time span, should never be routinely ordered (even if potassium levels are elevated) and are used only in acute cardiorespiratory arrest situations or to treat hyperkalemia-induced cardiac arrhythmias. Potassium values may drop quickly and to low levels, resulting in dangerous hypokalemic-induced arrhythmias.

- If sodium bicarbonate is used, it should be given by slow intravenous infusion over several hours. It should never be given as a bolus injection except in a cardiac arrest.

6 All patients with diabetic ketoacidosis need insulin.

A It takes longer to reverse the acidosis than to treat the hyperglycemia with insulin. Short-acting or rapid-acting insulin should always be used, producing relatively fast results in reducing glucose levels.

B Insulin treatment protocols may vary based on provider preference. However, a popular method to use is intravenous, low-dose, continuous infusion of insulin.

- The benefits of low-dose insulin infusions include a reduced risk of hypoglycemia and hypokalemia because decreases in glucose and potassium levels are predictable. Additionally, the theoretical risk of cerebral edema is decreased, and the need to estimate doses and administer repeated intramuscular injections is eliminated.

C An example of a protocol for giving a low-dose insulin infusion is shown in Figure 2.3.

7 Response to therapy can be predicted in most instances. Glucose levels should fall at the rate of approximately 75 to 100 mg/dL (4.2 to 5.6 mmol/L) per hour. Ketosis should be reversed in 12 to 24 hours, although occasionally urinary ketone bodies may be present for several days.

A The time-course for the reversal of acidosis has not been well studied because serial pH measurements are not carried out. However, as most patients recover from DKA, they experience a transient state of hyperchloremic acidosis.[5]

- Hyperchloremic acidosis is manifested by bicarbonate levels plateauing at approximately 15 to 20 mEq/L (15 to 20 mmol/L), usually between 12 to 24 hours after treatment is started.
- Chloride levels are elevated, pH has returned to normal, and serum ketone bodies are low or absent.
- The transient state does not require the administration of additional insulin, and recovery to a normal acid-base status occurs naturally.

B Overall mortality is less than 10%, with most deaths occurring in older patients primarily because of medical complications other than DKA.[6] Older age and depth of coma are the most accurate prognostic indicators. Death is usually due to infection, arterial thrombosis, or unrelenting shock.

- Even in the most controlled environment, complications in the treatment of DKA can occur. These complications can include aspiration, pulmonary edema, and unsuccessfully treated precipitating causes.
- Cerebral edema occurs rarely, but is the primary cause of death in children who succumb to DKA. When the patient's mental function begins to improve and then deteriorates while the metabolic condition continues to return to normal, cerebral edema should be suspected. One factor contributing to the development of cerebral edema may be that the rate of falling blood glucose levels is too rapid.
- The addition of intravenous glucose to the regimen is important once the serum glucose level reaches about 300 mg/dL (16.7 mmol/L).
- Treatment of cerebral edema, if it occurs, should include IV osmotic diuretics (mannitol) and possibly high-dose glucocorticoids (dexamethasone). The earlier the treatment, the better the prognosis.

Figure 2.3. Sample Approach for Low-Dose Insulin Infusion for DKA

1 Administer the insulin through a piggyback system into the existing intravenous (IV) line. It is preferable to use an infusion pump to assure accurate delivery of dosages.

2 Attach IV tubing and preflush with at least 50 mL of infusion to allow insulin to bind to the plastic tubing. This procedure ensures that the infusion entering the circulation contains the correct amount of insulin. It is not necessary to use albumin.

3 Some providers give 0.1 to 0.2 units/kg of body weight of regular insulin intravenously as a bolus. However, no benefit of this method has been documented.[9]

4 In children, give 0.1 to 0.2 units/kg of body weight of regular insulin per hour as a continuous infusion. In adults, the rate should be 5 to 10 units per hour as a continuous infusion.

5 The glucose level should drop approximately 75 to 100 mg/dL per hour with proper rehydration and insulin therapy. Administering insulin alone without appropriate fluid replacement will not be very effective in lowering glucose concentrations.

6 Monitor blood glucose levels after 1 hour and then every 1 to 2 hours. Double the insulin infusion rate if the glucose level has not dropped by 10% over 2 hours and the patient is being adequately hydrated. Check electrolyte values every 2 to 4 hours as needed. Because urinary ketone bodies may take several days to clear, their presence is not useful for management decisions. Serum ketone bodies measured by the nitroprusside method are also not helpful to chart the reversal of ketosis because ß-hydroxybutyrate is converted back to acetoacetate, which is the ketone body measured. Direct measurement of ß-hydroxybutyrate is now possible and may be helpful to monitor treatment.[10]

7 Subcutaneous insulin may be started when the patient is able to eat. Short-acting insulin should be given 30 minutes and rapid-acting insulin 15 minutes prior to discontinuing the IV insulin to maintain blood glucose in a safe range.

Source: Adapted from Davidson.[5]

8 Frequent errors made in the management of DKA include delay in diagnosis or misdiagnosis, delay in instituting therapy, and inadequate fluid replacement. Patients may be misdiagnosed as having gastroenteritis or appendicitis.

A Hypokalemia and cerebral edema may also go unrecognized, causing critical delays in beginning appropriate therapy for these conditions.

B It is essential to assess mental status frequently (every 1 to 2 hours), especially in children, who are more susceptible to cerebral edema than adults. Treatment of cerebral edema at early stages may be beneficial but is usually ineffective at later stages.

9 DKA can be prevented by thorough patient education, strategic planning, and rapid action (see Chapter 8, Illness and Surgery, in Diabetes Management Therapies, for more information on self-management guidelines for patients).

A Evaluate the patient's knowledge and sick-day management skills following an episode of DKA. Omitting insulin when unable to eat, not monitoring glucose levels frequently enough, and failing to test urine for ketones are common misjudgments. Ask the patient and family what they might specifically do differently next time. Review potential positive and negative consequences of actions they choose.

B A multidisciplinary team approach, including psychosocial intervention, is critical when caring for patients with recurrent episodes of DKA.

Hyperosmolar Hyperglycemic State

1 Hyperosmolar hyperglycemic state (HHS) is sometimes overlooked and often confused with other illnesses or conditions.

A HHS occurs in elderly patients with type 2 diabetes.

B HHS occurs in elderly patients who are being treated with medical nutrition therapy with or without oral antidiabetic agents and who may be inadequately monitored (eg, nursing home residents, those who live alone, elderly hospitalized patients who are not receiving adequate fluid intake or adequate monitoring of blood glucose and are often unable to communicate their needs). HHS is often precipitated by illness or other stresses. It can also be the initial presentation of type 2 diabetes.

C The symptoms that normally signal the onset of HHS may go unrecognized for several weeks in the elderly. The absence of significant ketosis (<2+ in a nitroprusside test in a 1:1 dilution of plasma) differentiates HHS from DKA.

D The mortality rate in HHS is greater than in DKA because of severe metabolic changes, delay in diagnosis, or other medical complications in elderly patients.

2 Some precipitating factors for HHS are massive fluid loss from prolonged osmotic diuresis secondary to hyperglycemia, severe burns, severe diarrhea, hemodialysis, peritoneal dialysis, and the use of thiazide or other diuretics.

A Other causes are infections, myocardial infarction, gastrointestinal hemorrhage, uremia, and arterial thrombosis.

B Hypertonic feeding (prolonged parenteral nutrition via IV infusion, high-protein or gastric tube feeding) and pharmacologic agents (eg, thiazides, propranolol, phenytoin, steroids, furosemide, chlorthalidone) may precipitate the onset of HHS.

Pathophysiology of HHS

1 HHS is considered to be a syndrome with 4 primary features: severe hyperglycemia, absence of significant ketosis, profound dehydration, and neurologic manifestations.

A HHS is similar to DKA except that insulin deficiency is probably less profound so increased lipolysis does not occur (Figure 2.1).

B Absence of ketosis and acidosis decreases gastrointestinal symptoms so that patients do not seek medical care as quickly. Consequently, the prolonged osmotic diuresis and dehydration secondary to hyperglycemia lead to decreased renal blood flow and allow glucose concentrations to reach a very high level.

C Impaired thirst mechanism or impaired ability to replace fluids, especially in the elderly, exacerbate the tendency toward HHS. Patients lose fluids over a longer time, so they may be more dehydrated than with DKA. Thus, blood urea nitrogen and creatinine levels may be higher.

D Because HHS patients are more dehydrated, mentation changes are more commonly seen than in DKA.

Signs and Symptoms of HHS

1 The signs and symptoms of HHS are similar to DKA, with several important exceptions. The gastrointestinal symptoms are usually milder than those found in DKA.

2 Kussmaul respirations are seldom observed because of a lack of severe acidosis.

3 Decreased mentation (eg, lethargy and mild confusion) is common in HHS. Frank coma is unusual. As in DKA, mentation correlates best with serum osmolality.

4 Patients with HHS may also have focal neurological signs (hemisensory deficits, hemiparesis, aphasia, and seizures) that mimic a cerebrovascular accident. These signs will abate as biochemical status is restored to normal. A comparison of DKA and HHS is shown in Table 2.2.

Initial Laboratory Values of HHS

1 Appropriate laboratory tests such as a complete blood cell count (CBC), roentgenogram, and cultures (blood, urine, and sputum) may help identify the precipitating cause of HHS.

2 The glucose level is usually >600 mg/dL (>33.3 mmol/L).

3 Ketone bodies are not present in the blood or urine except in small amounts.

4 Plasma osmolality is markedly elevated (usually >320 mOsm/kg).

Treatment of HHS

1 The primary treatment goal is rehydration to restore circulating plasma volume and correct electrolyte deficits. Additional treatment goals are similar to those for DKA:
  A Provide adequate insulin to restore and maintain normal glucose metabolism.
  B Prevent complications due to treatment of HHS.
  C Treat any underlying medical condition.
  D Provide patient/family education and follow-up.

Table 2.2. Diabetic Ketoacidosis (DKA) and Hyperosmolar Hyperglycemic State (HHS): Comparison of Some Salient Features

Feature	Conditions DKA	HHS
Age of patients	Usually <40 y	Usually >60 y
Duration of symptoms	Usually <2 d	Usually >5 d
Plasma glucose level	Usually <600 mg/dL (<33.3 mmol/L)	Usually >600 mg/dL (>33.3 mmol/L)
Sodium concentration	More likely to be normal or low	More likely to be normal or high
Potassium concentration	High, normal, or low	High, normal, or low
Bicarbonate concentration	Low	Normal
Ketone bodies	At least 4+ in 1:1 dilution	<2+ in 1:1 dilution
Arterial pH	Low	Normal
Serum osmolality	Often <320 m0sm/kg (<320 mmol/kg)	Usually >320 m0sm/kg (>320 mmol/kg)
Cerebral edema	Often subclinical; occasionally clinical	Subclinical has not been evaluated; rarely clinical
Prognosis	3% to 10% mortality	10% to 20% mortality
Subsequent course	Insulin therapy required in virtually all cases	Insulin therapy not required in many cases

Source: Adapted with permission from Davidson.[5]

2 Treatment is based on fluid and electrolyte replacement and administration of insulin.[1,11]

3 As in DKA, fluid replacement depends on the patient's state of hydration and cardiovascular status. Use caution when hydrating elderly patients to avoid fluid overload.

  A Because older patients are more likely to have a compromised cardiovascular status, fluid replacement with saline needs to be done cautiously.

  B Observe patients frequently to ensure that they are not developing congestive heart failure.

  C Patients with a previous history of cardiovascular disease should be monitored by central venous pressure or Swan-Ganz catheter.

4 Although glucose levels will not decrease appreciably without adequate rehydration, insulin administration is also an important treatment of HHS.

   A In general, the same guidelines for DKA apply.

   B Glucose and electrolyte levels need to be evaluated every 2 to 4 hours until they are stable.

   C Because treatment of acidosis is not part of HHS, insulin can be decreased when glucose values reach acceptable levels (~300 mg/dL [16.7 mmol/L]).[1]

5 To prevent HHS from occurring, identify high-risk patients, encourage adequate hydration, and educate patients and family about warning signs and symptoms.

   A Older adults need information about sick-day care.

   B Keep fluids within reach or offer fluids every 2 hours to hospital/nursing home residents.

Key Educational Considerations

1 The importance of recognizing the signs and symptoms of hyperglycemia, not omitting insulin, and maintaining adequate fluid intake need to be emphasized at diagnosis and reinforced regularly. Teach patients and their significant others when, whom, and how to call for help; reinforce this information frequently.

2 Effective teaching methods can include the use of analogies (particularly for explaining the physiology of the signs and symptoms) and the use of practice through simulation and situational problem solving.

3 Review the proper use of fluids (sugared and sugar-free), supplemental insulin when experiencing hyperglycemia and/or ketonemia, and blood glucose levels to serve as guidelines for "take-action" times.

4 After an acute episode of DKA or HHS, assess the patient and family's use of sick-day guidelines. Review specific precipitating factors and use the information to develop a plan with the patient to prevent reoccurrence. Children and adolescents who experience repeated episodes of DKA may need supervision of insulin injections.

5 Elderly patients (especially those living alone) may need to have a family member or friend check frequently for symptoms of hyperglycemia or a change in mentation to ensure prompt medical care if symptoms develop. Provide education to the patient and/or care provider about the risk, possible symptoms, and actions to take if the blood glucose rises to dangerous levels whenever patients are started on new medications that may exacerbate hyperglycemia.

Self-Review Questions

1 List the precipitating factors in the development of DKA.

2 Describe the pathophysiology of DKA.

3 List 3 presenting signs and symptoms of DKA.

4 What laboratory values indicate DKA?

5 List the 3 major treatment goals for DKA.

6 List the 2 precipitating factors of HHS.

7 Describe the pathophysiology of HHS.

8 List the presenting signs and symptoms of HHS.

9 What is the primary treatment for HHS?

10 What are 2 differences in laboratory values between DKA and HHS?

Learning Assessment: Case Study

CR is an 8-year-old female with known type 1 diabetes since the age of 6 years. She presents for her third admission to the ICU with a pH of 7.11, HCO_3 of 7, and blood glucose of 310 mg/dL. Over the past month, her healthcare team has continually recommended that her total daily insulin dose be increased, yet her blood glucose levels have remained in the 300 to 400 mg/dL range. She has continually had small to moderate ketones in her urine.

For the past week, CR has supplemented her usual insulin dose with an extra 3 to 4 units of rapid-acting insulin every 4 to 6 hours. Despite this additional insulin, her urine showed large ketones at the time of admission. Her oral intake of food and fluids has been increasingly poor over the 3 days prior to arrival. Insulin was omitted on the day of admission because she had no oral intake that day. Her parents report no emesis at home, but she did have 1 episode of large emesis on arrival to the emergency room. Her only physical complaint was abdominal pain. Her parents report there has been no change in her usual meal-planning patterns. She has been administering her own insulin injections, despite a request by the diabetes educator for the parents to do so.

The physical exam reveals a temperature of 36.3°C, pulse 140, respirations 25 and slightly labored, BP 137/69, and a weight of 59 lb (26.8 kg) (down from 27.9 kg 14 days prior). Her lips and mucosa are dry, and the rest of the exam is unremarkable.

Questions for Discussion

1 How should treatment proceed?

2 What interventions could the diabetes care team initiate?

3 What are possible reasons for CR's DKA?

Discussion

1 History and symptoms are classic for DKA.

2 An IV was started and CR was given an infusion of D5/.45 normal saline solution with 20 mEq/L potassium chloride and 20 mEq/L potassium phosphate at a rate of 67 cc/hour. An additional infusion of one half normal saline was run at 33 cc/hour.

3 An insulin infusion was begun at a rate of 3 units/hour.

4 Blood glucose levels and electrolyte levels were checked hourly, and the insulin drip and IVs were adjusted accordingly. On the day following admission, CR's blood glucose level normalized. The insulin drip was continued until adequate hydration and oral intake were established.

5 CR then started to eat her usual meal plan. Subcutaneous insulin administration was initiated 30 minutes prior to discontinuing the insulin drip and the dose was adjusted over the next several days.

6 During her hospital stay, CR and her parents met with the diabetes nurse and the dietitian. Since both of CR's parents expressed frustration about CR's insulin routine and the many hospitalizations, along with the concern that CR was not receiving all of her prescribed insulin, the opportunity to consult with a psychologist was offered.

7 The following suggestions were offered to help prevent future hospitalizations: continue to monitor blood glucose closely, explore reasons for parental reluctance to give insulin injections, and call daily for further insulin dose adjustment and problem solving. Further discussions with CR and her parents are also needed. Ask CR's parents what they believe to be the cause of her DKA and what they are willing to do to prevent future occurrences. Asking CR what it is like for her at home and school might provide insights about possible precipitating factors.

8 Outpatient follow-up was scheduled with the diabetes team 2 weeks following hospital discharge.

9 CR's saga is a typical one. Recurrent episodes of DKA are not the norm in children with diabetes and are often related to omission of insulin injections. Most often, when there are repeated episodes, the diabetes educator needs to assess for a psychosocial etiology. Children often "like" being in the hospital; when they are "ill," their parents give them undivided attention and concern. However, repeated DKA episodes can have disastrous outcomes. CR will need the support of her diabetes care team, including her parents, on an ongoing basis if further episodes of DKA are to be prevented.

References

1 American Diabetes Association. Hyperglycemic crises in patients with diabetes mellitus (position statement). Diabetes Care. 2001;24(Suppl 1):S83-S90.

2 The Expert Committee on the Diagnosis and Classification of Diabetes Mellitus. Report of the expert committee on the diagnosis and classification of diabetes mellitus. Diabetes Care. 2001;24(Suppl 1):S5-S20.

3 Marshall SM, George K, Alberti MM. Hyperosmolar hyperglycemic nonketotic coma. In: DeFronzo RA, ed. Current Therapy of Diabetes Mellitus. St. Louis: Mosby, 1998:27.

4 DeFronzo RA, Matsuda M, Barrett EJ. Diabetic ketoacidosis: a combined metabolic nephrologic approach to therapy. Diabetes Rev. 1994;2:204-238.

5 Davidson MB. Diabetic ketoacidosis and hyperosmolar nonketotic coma. In: Davidson MB, ed. Diabetes Mellitus: Diagnosis and Treatment. 4th ed. New York: WB Saunders Company; 1998:159-194.

6 Siperstein MD. Diabetic ketoacidosis and hyperosmolar coma. Endocrinol Metab Clin North Am. 1992;21:415-432.

7 Lebovitz HE. Diabetic ketoacidosis. Lancet. 1995;345:767-772.

8 Glaser N, Barnett P, McCaslin I, et al for the Pediatric Emergency Medicine Collaborative Research Committee of the American Academy of Pediatrics. Risk factors for cerebral edema in children with diabetic ketoacidosis. N Engl J Med. 2001;344:264-269.

9 Krane EJ. Diabetic ketoacidosis and cerebral edema on the Internet. Available at: *http://pedsccm.wusl.edu/FILE-CAB-INET/Metab/DKA-Cedema.html.* Accessed 1998.

10 Wiggam MI, O'Kane MJ, Harper R, et al. Treatment of diabetic ketoacidosis using normalization of blood 3-hydroxybutyrate concentration as the endpoint of emergency management. Diabetes Care. 1997;20:1347-1352.

11 Genuth S. Diabetic ketoacidosis and hyperosmolar hyperglycemic nonketotic syndrome in adults. In: Lebovitz HE, ed. Therapy for Diabetes Mellitus and Related Disorders. 3rd ed. Alexandria, Va: American Diabetes Association; 1998:90-95.

Suggested Readings

American Diabetes Association. Hyperglycemic crises in patients with diabetes mellitus (position statement). Diabetes Care. 2001;24(Suppl 1):S83-S90.

DeFronzo RA, Matsuda M, Barrett EJ. Diabetic ketoacidosis: a combined metabolic nephrologic approach to therapy. Diabetes Rev. 1994;2:204-238.

Ennis ED, Stahl EJVB, Kreisberg RA. The hyperosmolar hyperglycemic nonketotic syndrome. Diabetes Rev. 1994;1:115-126.

Foster DW, McGarry JD. The metabolic derangement and treatment of diabetic ketoacidosis. N Engl J Med. 1983;309:159-169.

Hinnen D, Childs B. Diabetes ketoacidosis and hyperosmolar nonketotic coma. In: Bucher L, Melander S, eds. Critical Care Nursing. Philadelphia: WB Saunders Company; 1999.

Kitabchi AE, Umpierrez GE, Murphy MB, et al. Management of hyperglycemic crises in patients with diabetes mellitus (technical review). Diabetes Care. 2001;224:131-153.

Kaufman FR, Halvorsen M. The treatment and prevention of diabetic ketoacidosis in children and adolescents with type 1 diabetes. Pediatr Annals. 1999;28:576-582.

Learning Assessment: Post-Test Questions

Hyperglycemia

1   Prolonged hyperglycemia from uncontrolled diabetes mellitus can lead to 1 of 2 metabolic crises. They are:
    A   Ketoacidosis and hyperosmolar hyperglycemic state
    B   Diabetic neuritis and hyperosmolar hypertension
    C   Cerebral vascular accident and severe dehydration
    D   Diabetic nephrosis and acute dehydration

2   Which of the following is not likely to be a precipitating factor in the development of diabetic ketoacidosis?
    A   Illness or infection
    B   Insufficient insulin
    C   Hypertension
    D   Emotional stress

3   HHS is a life-threatening emergency with high mortality rate. It is often seen in which type of patients?
    A   Middle-aged type 1
    B   Youthful type 2
    C   Teenage gestational
    D   Elderly type 2

4   A prominent respiratory symptom present in diabetic ketoacidosis is:
    A   Shallow breathing
    B   Deep respirations
    C   Wheezing
    D   Hypoventilation

5   During HHS and DKA, mental function is most directly affected by:
    A   Plasma sodium level
    B   Serum osmolality
    C   Degree of acidosis
    D   Hyperglycemia

6   The reason the outcome of diabetic ketoacidosis is frequently less severe than that of HHS is that:
    A   A person experiencing DKA frequently receives medical help when symptoms first appear
    B   DKA generally occurs among older adults who are more likely to take better care of themselves
    C   A person has some insulin reserves that tend to blunt symptoms
    D   A person is not likely to lose consciousness during a DKA episode

7   During acidosis, the serum bicarbonate concentration, blood pH, and carbon dioxide pressure will be:
    A   Elevated
    B   Lower
    C   Unchanged
    D   Variable

8   Patients with HHS may have focal neurological signs that mimic:
    A   Myocardial infarction
    B   Diabetic ketoacidosis
    C   Multiple sclerosis
    D   Cerebral vascular accident

9   Which of the following features is not present in HHS?
    A   Severe hyperglycemia
    B   Neurologic manifestations
    C   Presence of ketosis
    D   Profound dehydration

10 The immediate treatment goal for diabetic ketoacidosis is to:
    A   Assess and correct fluid and electrolyte imbalance
    B   Provide education and follow-up with the family
    C   Diminish insulin administration and acidosis
    D   Prevent long-term degenerative complications

11 A person has been admitted to the emergency room with the following symptoms: severe hyperglycemia (>800 mg/dL), absence of ketoacidosis, profound dehydration, and neurologic signs ranging from depressed sensorium to coma. What life-threatening emergency may be occurring?

A Diabetic ketoacidosis

B Hyperosmolar hyperglycemic state

C Cerebral vascular accident

D Chronic obstructive pulmonary disease

12 Kussmaul respirations are the physiologic response to:

A Metabolic alkalosis

B Dehydration

C Metabolic acidosis

D Hypotension

13 Which is the most accurate statement regarding the sodium concentration?

A If the deficit of sodium is greater than that of water, the sodium level will be high

B If the deficit of sodium is greater than that of water, the sodium level will be low

C If the deficit of sodium is greater than that of water, the 2 deficiencies will be roughly equal

D The sodium level does not correspond to the H_2O level

See next page for answer key.

Post-Test Answer Key

Hyperglycemia 2

1	A		8	D
2	C		9	C
3	D		10	A
4	B		11	B
5	B		12	C
6	A		13	B
7	B			

A Core Curriculum for Diabetes Education
Diabetes and Complications

Chronic Complications of Diabetes: An Overview   3

Mindy Andrus, RD, LDN, CDE
Nancy Leggett-Frazier RN, MSN, CDE
Michael A. Pfeifer, MD, FACE, CDE
East Carolina University
Brody School of Medicine
Greenville, North Carolina

Introduction

1 Chronic complications of diabetes were virtually unknown until 10 to 20 years after the discovery of insulin in 1921.

   A Descriptions of renal disease, neuropathy, and retinopathy did not appear until the 1930s and 1940s. At that time, it was not clear whether these complications (especially the microvascular abnormalities) were an integral part of diabetes mellitus or a consequence of poor blood glucose control.

   B Studies such as the Diabetes Control and Complications Trial (DCCT)[1] among individuals with type 1 diabetes and the United Kingdom Prospective Diabetes Study (UKPDS)[2] among individuals with type 2 diabetes have demonstrated that these complications are not inevitable.

2 This chapter will enumerate both the modifiable and nonmodifiable risk factors of diabetes complications to provide the background for the content in each complication-specific chapter and to assist educators to present this information to persons with diabetes in a meaningful way.

3 The diabetes educator can play a key role in the prevention of chronic complications by providing information to patients about behaviors and nonpharmacologic options that may affect their development.

4 Education concerning the reduction of modifiable risk factors for the chronic complications of diabetes is an essential component of diabetes self-management education. Although the influence of hyperglycemia has become part of standard diabetes self-management education, other risk factors have often received less attention.

5 Persons with diabetes need information about risk factors that may increase chronic complications in order to make informed decisions and fully participate in their own care.

6 The chronic complications of diabetes significantly impact the cost of health care. Approximately 25% of the total Medicare budget is dedicated to the treatment of diabetes and its chronic complications.[3] It has been estimated that by reducing or eliminating risk factors, 85% of the chronic complications could be delayed or the progression slowed. This would save the Medicare budget more than $17 billion annually.

7 The pathogenesis of diabetes complications has been studied for the last 50 years. No single etiology explains all of the complications; rather, multiple etiologies exist that are specific to each.

   A Hyperglycemia plays a role in the etiology of all complications; there are also additional risk factors associated with each, resulting in complex, and perhaps independent, etiologies. Glucose goals for people with diabetes are listed in Table 3.1.

   B The etiology of complications is further confounded by the variation in risk factors among individuals. In some individuals, one or more risk factors may play a greater role than in other individuals.

Table 3.1 Glycemic Control for People With Diabetes*

	Normal	Goal	Additional Action Suggested†
Whole blood values			
Average preprandial glucose (mg/dL)‡	<100	80 to 120	<80/>140
Average bedtime glucose (mg/dL)‡	<110	100 to 140	<100/>160
Plasma values			
Average preprandial glucose (mg/dL)**	<110	90 to 130	<90/>150
Average bedtime glucose (mg/dL)**	<120	110 to 150	<110/>180
A1C (%) ‡‡	<6	<7	>8

* The values in this table are by necessity generalized to the entire population of individuals with diabetes. Patients with comorbid diseases, the very young and older adults, and others with unusual conditions or circumstances may warrant different treatment goals. These values are for nonpregnant adults.

† "Additional action suggested" depends on the individual patient circumstances. Such actions may include enhanced diabetes self-management education, comanagement with a diabetes team, referral to an endocrinologist, changes in pharmacological therapies, or more frequent contact with the patient.

‡ Measurement of capillary blood glucose.

** Values calibrated to plasma glucose.

‡‡ A1C is referenced to a nondiabetic range of 4.0% to 6.0%.

Source: Reprinted with permission from the American Diabetes Association.[4]

The American Association of Clinical Endocrinologists (ACE) recommends a primary target glucose goal of A1C <6.5%, a target fasting plasma glucose of <100 mg/dL, and a target 2-hour postmeal glucose of <140 mg/dL.[5]

    C Determining which risk factor carries the greatest possibility for the development of each complication, as well as the variation among individuals, has been an area of intense investigation.

8 Pathophysiologic mechanisms which are hypothesized to contribute to the development of specific complications include

    A Accumulation of intracellular sorbitol from the conversion of glucose to sorbitol *(polyol pathway)*

    B Autoimmunity

    C Tissue ischemia and hypoxia

    D Glycosylation of cellular proteins *(advanced glycosylated end products [AGE])*

    E Coagulation defects

    F Insulin resistance

Objectives

Upon completion of this chapter, the learner will be able to

1 State the modifiable risk factors for individuals with diabetes for cardiovascular disease, neuropathy, nephropathy, and retinopathy.

2 State the nonmodifiable risk factors for persons with diabetes for cardiovascular disease, neuropathy, nephropathy, and retinopathy.

3 State glucose, lipid, and blood pressure goals for people with diabetes.

4 Describe the impact of hyperglycemia on the long-term complications of diabetes.

Cardiovascular Complications

1 Macrovascular complications include coronary artery disease, myocardial infarction, peripheral vascular disease, and cerebral vascular disease (see Chapter 6, Macrovascular Disease, in Diabetes and Complications, for more information).

2 Nonmodifiable risk factors include duration of diabetes, age, genetics, race, and gender.
  A A linear relationship appears to exist between the duration of diabetes and cardiovascular complications. This relationship may be more observable in individuals with type 1 diabetes, since the onset of type 2 diabetes is not easily established.
  B As in individuals without diabetes, there is a relationship between age and the prevalence of cardiovascular disease. The older the individual with diabetes, the greater the risk for cardiovascular complications.
  C Genetics play a role in the incidence of cardiovascular complications, although predictive genetic characteristics have not been fully elucidated.
  D African-American individuals with diabetes are at risk for macrovascular disease, but have an overall lower prevalence rate of myocardial infarction (MI) than Caucasian individuals.[6] Mexican-American individuals appear to have an increased risk for peripheral vascular disease, but a lower prevalence of MI than Caucasian individuals.[7]
  E Premenopausal women without diabetes are at less risk than males without diabetes for cardiovascular events and complications. This gender-protective advantage does not exist for females with diabetes, who have an equal risk for cardiovascular events and complications as males with diabetes.[8]

3 Modifiable risk factors include hyperglycemia, hypertension, dyslipidemia, increased platelet adherence, smoking, eating habits, increased homocysteine level, obesity, increased insulin level, lack of exercise, and type A personality.
  A The evidence suggests that treatment of hyperglycemia will result in a decrease in cardiovascular events or complications, but is not conclusive. The DCCT data were suggestive (45% to 54% reduction) but did not reach statistical significance regarding this relationship.[1] The UKPDS also showed this relationship, but again did not quite reach statistical significance.[2] A Finnish study did conclude that metabolic control of type 2 diabetes and duration of diabetes are important predictors of coronary heart disease in the elderly, particularly among women.[9] Nonetheless, improved glucose control will decrease total cholesterol levels, decrease LDL cholesterol, and decrease platelet adherence.
  B Hypertension appears to play a major role in the development of cardiovascular complications in individuals with diabetes as well as individuals without diabetes.[10]
    • Hypertension is twice as common in African-American individuals than in Caucasian individuals with diabetes.[6]

- Hypertension prevalence increases with age among people with diabetes. A larger percentage of individuals with diabetes have hypertension than do age-comparable individuals without diabetes.
- An increase in vascular response to stimuli may play a role in hypertension in diabetes.
- Hyperinsulinemia, theoretically, might play a role by increasing the tubular reabsorption of sodium and thereby increasing blood volume.
- The primary goal of therapy for blood pressure for adults should be to decrease blood pressure to <130/80 mm Hg. In children, blood pressure should be decreased to the corresponding age-adjusted 90th percentile values.[4]

C Dyslipidemia involves 4 major areas of concern for individuals with diabetes: decreased high-density lipoprotein cholesterol level (HDL), increased low-density lipoprotein (LDL) cholesterol level, increased triglyceride (TG) level, and increased lipoprotein Lp(a) level.[11] Lipid goals are listed in Table 3.2.[4]

Table 3.2. Lipid Goals for Adults With Diabetes

	Goal
Cholesterol	<200 mg/dL (5.17 mmol/L)
LDL cholesterol	<100 mg/dL (2.6 mmol/L)
HDL cholesterol	Men: >45 mg/dL (1.15 mmol/L) Women: >55 mg/dL (1.40 mmol/L)
Triglycerides	<150 mg/dL (1.7 mmol/L)

Source: Reprinted with permission from the American Diabetes Association.[4]

D People with diabetes can have an increase in platelet adherence and aggregation that may lead to abnormalities in microcirculation and add to plaque formation. Improved metabolic control has been shown to decrease platelet adherence and aggregation.[12,13]

E The link between smoking and cardiovascular events and complications is well established in individuals with or without diabetes. The benefits of smoking cessation have been demonstrated in nondiabetic populations. There is no reason to believe that smoking cessation would not be beneficial for individuals with diabetes.[14,15]

F Diets high in fat have been suggested to increase atherosclerosis via increased plasma cholesterol, in particular, LDL cholesterol levels. There is controversy, however, whether educational and nutritional efforts should be directed towards a very low-fat composition versus a low saturated fat/high monounsaturated fat composition. However, the need to decrease intake of foods containing saturated fat, because it increases LDL cholesterol, is clear.[16] Furthermore, preliminary evidence suggests that a diet high in total fat may contribute to insulin resistance.[17]

G Homocystine is increased only in individuals with diabetes and vascular disease or retinopathy. Elevated homocystine levels may cause tears in the endothelium. No prospective studies have been conducted demonstrating that a decrease in homocystine level results in decreased cardiovascular events. Homocystine levels may be decreased by pharmacological doses of pyridoxine (vitamin B_6), vitamin B_{12}, and folic acid.[18]

H Obesity, particularly central adiposity, has been linked to atherogenesis. However, no prospective, randomized clinical trial has shown that a decrease in adiposity will decrease cardiovascular events. Because increased adiposity is linked with hypertension, dyslipidemia, hyperinsulinemia, and hyperglycemia, it seems prudent that a decrease in adiposity would contribute to decreasing cardiovascular events.

I Increased insulin levels have been linked to both hypertension and atherosclerosis in cross-sectional data in nondiabetic populations,[12] leading to a suggestion that insulin resistance is associated with increased cardiovascular risks. However, no data indicating that insulin is atherogenic in humans are available.

J Lack of exercise is associated with cardiovascular events and complications. Routine exercise decreases blood pressure, often decreases blood glucose levels, is important for cardiac toning, and is useful as a way to cope with stress and as an adjunct to weight loss. There are few data that link the benefits of exercise to prolongation of life after myocardial infarction. Cross-sectional epidemiologic and anecdotal data suggest that a routine exercise program can help prevent cardiovascular events in patients who have not had a myocardial infarction.[19,20]

K Individuals with a Type A (high strung) personality are at increased risk for cardiovascular events and their complications.[21] Psychological and behavioral therapies have been shown to decrease cardiovascular events in individuals without diabetes. This benefit is thought to be realized by individuals with diabetes as well.

4 Other risk factors include plasminogen activator inhibitor 1, Von Willebrand factor, fibrinogen, fibrinolysis, and microcirculation. All of these factors have been linked, in cross-sectional studies in animals, to increased cardiovascular events, suggesting they may also play a role in humans with diabetes. However, convincing prospective studies are lacking.

5 The following are characteristics not believed to be risk factors for cardiovascular complications.

A The type of diabetes does not appear to be a factor in the development of cardiovascular disease. However, cardiovascular events and complications occur with higher frequency in individuals with type 2 diabetes than in individuals with type 1 diabetes. Persons with type 1 diabetes develop cardiovascular disease at a younger age than nondiabetic persons.

B There is no known evidence of an autoimmune process causing cardiovascular complications in individuals with diabetes.

Neuropathy

1 Diabetic neuropathy includes distal symmetrical polyneuropathy, autonomic neuropathy, mononeuropathies, plexopathies, proximal motor neuropathy, and entrapment neuropathies (see Chapter 9, Neuropathy, in Diabetes and Complications, for more information).

2 Nonmodifiable risk factors include duration of diabetes, age, genetics, race, height, and autoimmunity.

A There is a linear relationship between the duration of diabetes and the development of diabetic neuropathy; the longer one has diabetes, the greater the risk of developing diabetic neuropathy.

B Age also appears to be related in a linear fashion to the development of diabetic neuropathy; older age in a person with diabetes is associated with a greater likelihood that neuropathy will develop.

C Diabetic neuropathy is influenced by genetics; human leukocyte antigens (HLA) DR3 and DR4 have been linked to an increased incidence of this complication.[22]

D African Americans are more likely to develop diabetic neuropathy than Caucasians.[23,24]

E Taller individuals tend to have more diabetic neuropathy than shorter individuals, possibly due to the length of the nerve and the increased probability of abnormalities due to this length.[25] Although in a recent study,[26] increasing height was not associated with neuropathy severity.

F *Autoimmunity* involves the body's antibodies attacking itself in an unwanted assault, in this case, against the nerves. There is an increase in the level of autoantibodies to nerves in some individuals with diabetes and neuropathy.[27] It is not clear whether the autoantibodies are a response to damaged nerves or the autoantibodies cause the damage. Thus, it is not clear whether this is a primary etiology in the development of neuropathy. Once autoantibodies are formed, they hasten the progression of the diabetic neuropathy.

3 Modifiable risk factors include hyperglycemia, hypertension, dyslipidemia, abnormal microcirculation, and alcohol use.

A Hyperglycemia may play several roles in the development of diabetic neuropathy.
  - Hyperglycemia may cause an increased incidence of glycosylated neural proteins and formation of advanced glycosylated end products (AGEs). Such alterations of the neural proteins may decrease nerve transport and affect protein function.
  - Hyperglycemia can competitively inhibit the uptake of myoinositol by the nerve. Myoinositol is important for nerve membrane function and maintaining the Na-K-TPase activity.
  - Hyperglycemia can activate the polyol pathway, leading to increased concentration of sorbitol within the nerve. This, in turn, can cause swelling within the space between the nerve fibers (endoneuria) within the nerve sheath, which can damage the nerve and alter nerve function. In addition, activation of the polyol pathway may decrease nerve myoinositol through unknown mechanisms.
  - Hyperglycemia can decrease nitric oxide synthetase activity, which, in turn, may decrease microcirculation to the nerve.
  - Insulin deficiency may retard the conversion of the fatty acid linoleic acid to gamma-linoleic acid. This may cause a deviation in prostaglandin pathways, causing a decrease in the formation of arachidonic acid. This decrease in arachidonic acid alters the constituents of the nerve membrane.

B Hypertension,[23] particularly the diastolic level, is linked to the development of diabetic neuropathy. This finding is consistent in several correctional studies including the DCCT.[1] At least one study[28] has shown an increase in nerve conduction velocity when patients were placed on an angiotensin-converting enzyme (ACE) inhibitor.

C Hypercholesterolemia is associated with the development of diabetic neuropathy. However, no prospective studies have shown that a decrease in cholesterol levels will decrease the onset or slow the progression of diabetic neuropathy.

D The relationship between heavy alcohol ingestion and an increased incidence of neuropathy has been demonstrated.[29] Alcohol alone can cause nerve damage. Combining the effects of alcohol with the nerve damage due to diabetes may worsen the overall clinical picture.

4 Characteristics not believed to be risk factors for neuropathy.

A There are no data to suggest that the type of antidiabetes medications predisposes patients to, nor protects patients from, diabetic neuropathy.

B Males were once thought to be at greater risk for developing diabetic neuropathy than females.[30] However, considering that males are generally taller than females, it is felt that it is the height of the individual, not the gender, that predisposes individuals to develop diabetic neuropathy.

C There is no evidence to suggest that specific diets may predispose patients to diabetic neuropathy. Conversely, a diet high in myoinositol has been shown to increase nerve conduction velocity.[31]

D Neither increased nor decreased adiposity has been linked to the development of, or protection from, diabetic neuropathy.

E Exercise does not seem to play a role in the development of, or protection from, diabetic neuropathy. Exercise may put the insensate foot at risk for traumatic injury resulting in diabetic foot ulcers.

F There is no evidence to suggest a relationship between increased insulin levels and increased incidence of diabetic neuropathy.

G Some studies[24,32] have indicated that there is a cross-sectional relationship between smoking and diabetic neuropathy; however, this relationship has not been universally found.

Foot Ulcers

1 Foot ulcers develop primarily as a consequence of vascular disease, various types of neuropathies, foot deformities, or other factors affecting the health of the foot. Each of these causative factors has specific modifiable or nonmodifiable risk factors (see Chapter 4, Diabetic Foot Care and Education, in Diabetes and Complications, for more information).

2 Peripheral vascular disease plays a major role in the development of foot ulcers.

3 Neuropathy plays an essential role in the development of diabetic foot ulcers.

A An insensate foot puts the patient at increased risk for traumatic damage without an awareness of the injury. As a result, proper attention and care is often not sought in a timely manner.

B Autonomic dysfunction of the sweat glands of the foot may cause the skin to become dry and cracked and prone to ulceration.

C Patients with diabetic neuropathy often have motor abnormalities which may predispose them to trauma secondary to an unsteady gait and falls secondary to lack of proprioception (awareness of where the foot is in space).

D Neuropathy in the muscular part of the foot, leading to foot deformities and increased pressure points, may predispose the foot to ulcers. The metatarsal heads, interdigital joints, and tips of toes particularly are at high risk for development of foot ulcers from neuropathic muscular changes.

4 Amputation rates are higher among African Americans,[5] Hispanics,[6] and Native Americans[33] than Caucasians.

5 Exercise may predispose the insensate foot to traumatic damage if it is done in an imprudent manner. Choosing activities that avoid repeated pounding to the feet (swimming, bicycling) may be more prudent than jogging.

6 Other risk factors include improperly fitting shoes and nail abnormalities, visual impairments, lack of self-management skills.

Nephropathy

1 Diabetes is the most common cause of nephropathy. It is also, at present, the most costly complication of diabetes, due to the success of renal dialysis and kidney transplants. Early evidence of nephropathy is determined by the presence of albumin in urine. As the disease progresses, the amount of albumin increases until end-stage renal disease is reached (see Chapter 8, Nephropathy, in Diabetes and Complications, for more information).

2 Nonmodifiable risk factors include duration of diabetes, age, genetics, and race.
   A A relationship between duration of diabetes and end-stage renal disease is well established in individuals with type 1 diabetes but not in individuals with type 2 diabetes, partly because the onset of type 2 diabetes is seldom well documented.
   - The natural history (clinical stages) of nephropathy is thought to be the same in type 1 and in type 2 diabetes. See Table 3.3 for definitions of abnormalities in albumin excretion.[4]
   - Generally, end-stage renal disease occurs between 10 to 25 years' duration of diabetes. There is a decline in the prevalence of end-stage renal disease after 25 to 30 years' duration, although the risk is not totally eliminated.
   B A linear relationship exists between age and the development of diabetic nephropathy. The older the individual, the greater the risk of developing nephropathy.
   C Certain human leukocyte antigen (HLA) types are associated with the development of diabetic nephropathy.[34]
   D African Americans,[5] Hispanics,[6] and Native Americans[33] all have a greater prevalence of diabetic nephropathy than Caucasians with diabetes.

3 Modifiable risk factors include hypertension, dyslipidemia, hyperglycemia, eating habits, smoking, and frequent urinary tract infections.
   A The effect of hypertension on the development of nephropathy in individuals with diabetes or without diabetes is well documented.[34]
   - There is some evidence that treatment with certain antihypertensive agents may reduce the incidence or slow the progression of nephropathy. In particular, ACE inhibitors decrease blood pressure (that is, reduce pressure going into the glomeruli) as well as reduce resistance within the glomeruli.

Table 3.3. Definitions of Abnormalities of Albumin Excretion

	24-h Collection, mg/24 h	Timed Collection, µg/min	Spot Collection, µg/mg creatinine
Normal	<30	<20	<30
Microalbuminuria	30 to 299	20 to 199	30 to 299
Macroalbuminuria	≥300	≥200	≥300

Because of variability in urinary albumin excretion, 2 of 3 specimens collected within a 3- to 6-month period should be abnormal before considering a patient to have crossed one of these diagnostic thresholds. Exercise within 24 hours, infection, fever, congestive heart failure, marked hyperglycemia, and marked hypertension may elevate urinary albumin excretion over baseline values.

Source: Reprinted with permission from American Diabetes Association.[4]

- In prospective trials,[35] the ACE inhibitor captopril has been shown to increase the time to reach a doubling of the serum creatinine level, thus slowing the progression to end-stage renal disease.

B Cross-sectional studies[36] have linked hypercholesterolemia to the presence of diabetic nephropathy.

- In prospective trials,[37] treatment with HMG-CoA reductase inhibitor antilipidemia agents ("statin" drugs such as pravastatin, lovastatin, atorvastatin, fluvastatin, simvastatin, cerivastatin) has been shown to decrease cholesterol levels and increase the time to doubling of the serum creatinine level compared with the placebo group.

C Hyperglycemia may play several roles in the development of diabetic nephropathy.

- Hyperglycemia can lead to *glycosylation* (increased amount of glucose molecules attaching to proteins) of glomerular proteins and the formation of advanced glycation end products (AGEs). The development of AGEs results in protein structural changes, which can alter protein function.

- Hyperglycemia can result in activation of the polyol pathway. Accumulation of sorbitol produced by increased activity of the polyol pathway has been demonstrated in the glomeruli. This may lead to a decrease in glomerular function and allow micro quantities of albumin to leak into the urine *(microalbuminuria)*.

D There is little evidence that a high-protein diet results in the development of diabetic nephropathy or that a low-protein diet prevents the development of diabetic nephropathy.[38] However, once diabetic nephropathy develops, the rate of progression of the nephropathy can be slowed by placing the patient on a low-protein diet.[39]

E Cross-sectional studies[40] have linked smoking to the presence of diabetic nephropathy. No prospective trials have been done.

F Frequent urinary tract infections predispose a patient to glomerulonephritis and papillary necrosis, thus worsening existing renal dysfunction.

4 Certain characteristics are not believed to be risk factors.

  A There is no evidence that the type of antidiabetes treatment protects or predisposes an individual to diabetic nephropathy. However, metformin is contraindicated in renal disease because of the elimination profile of the drug.

  B There is no evidence that gender protects or predisposes an individual to the development of diabetic nephropathy.

  C Cross-sectional or prospective data are not available to document autoimmunity as a possible pathogenesis.

  D Strenuous exercise can increase proteinuria but there is no evidence of long-term damaging effects provided the patient does not have clinical evidence of renal disease.[41] There is no evidence that exercise helps slow the progression of diabetic nephropathy.

  E There is no evidence that adiposity is either protective or predisposes a patient for diabetic nephropathy.

  F There is no evidence that increased insulin levels are associated with the development of diabetic nephropathy.

Retinopathy

1 Diabetic retinopathy is the leading cause of blindness in the US and has been the focus of several large, multicenter, double-blind, randomized clinical trials. *Diabetic retinopathy* is described by the changes that occur in the retina, including microaneurysms, hard exudates, soft exudates, hemorrhages, and peripheral retinopathy (see Chapter 7, Eye Disease and Adaptive Education for Visually Impaired Persons, for more information).

2 Nonmodifiable risk factors include duration of diabetes, age, genetics, and race.

  A Duration of diabetes is linked to the development of retinopathy in type 1 diabetes.[42] A similar relationship is believed to exist for type 2 diabetes, but is not as well understood.

  - There is seldom a need for laser therapy within the first 10 years' duration of diabetes; laser therapy is most often needed between 10 and 22 years' duration of diabetes.[43]
  - There is a small increase in the need for laser therapy after 22 years' of duration of diabetes.
  - Some diabetic retinopathy is present in 90% of patients with diabetes by 20 years' disease duration.

  B There is a linear relationship between age and prevalence of diabetic retinopathy.

  C Diabetic retinopathy is influenced by genetics; human leukocyte antigens (HLA) DR3 and DR4 predispose for the development of this complication more than other HLA types.[44]

  D African Americans and Hispanics[5,6] are more likely to develop diabetic retinopathy than Caucasians. Retinopathy has also been reported in many Native American tribes.[33]

3 Modifiable risk factors include hyperglycemia, hypertension, dyslipidemia, abnormal microcirculation, and smoking.

A The development and progression of retinopathy correlates strongly with the degree of glycemic control.[1,2]

- One mechanism may be hyperglycemia-activation of the polyol pathway in the pericytes. The pericytes are the first cells to become abnormal and "pericyte ghosts" are formed early in the development of diabetic retinopathy. As a result, leakage (hard exudates) of albumin occur within the retina. In addition, outpouching of the capillary walls (microaneurysms) develop as a result of pericyte loss.

B Hypertension clearly plays a role in the development of diabetic retinopathy. Current data[45] suggest that ACE inhibitors may be particularly effective in slowing the progression of diabetic retinopathy.

C High cholesterol levels have been linked to the development of diabetic retinopathy in cross-sectional studies.[42] No prospective studies have been done.

D Areas of microischemia and microinfarctions (soft exudates) produce areas of hypoxia. As a result, there is increased formation of new blood vessels. However, the vessels are not well supported because of the vitreous fluid. These vessels are often very fragile and susceptible to bleeding, resulting in hemorrhage.

E Smoking has been linked to the development of retinopathy. Prospective randomized studies have not been performed.

4 Certain characteristics are not believed to be risk factors

A To date, there are no data concerning whether the type of antidiabetes treatment protects or predisposes individuals to diabetic retinopathy.

B There are very few data concerning whether gender protects or predisposes an individual to the development of diabetic retinopathy.

C The type of diabetes does not protect an individual from diabetic retinopathy; persons with all types of diabetes may develop retinopathy. However, the incidence of proliferative retinopathy is greater in type 1 than in type 2 diabetes.

D Although the predisposing human leukocyte antigen (HLA) types may imply an autoimmune basis, no autoantibodies have been identified to date.

E Eating habits do not appear to be protective nor predisposing to diabetic retinopathy.

F Some studies[42] have demonstrated that increased adiposity is associated with the presence of retinopathy. However, this association has not been universally found.

G There is no evidence that increased insulin levels influence the incidence of diabetic retinopathy.

H For patients who have proliferative diabetic retinopathy that is active, strenuous activity may precipitate vitreous hemorrhage or traction retinal detachment. Anaerobic exercise and any exercise that involves straining, jarring, or Valsalva-like maneuvers should be avoided[41] (see Chapter 2, Exercise, in Diabetes Management Therapies, for more information).

Other Long-Term Concerns or Issues

1 Certain long-term problems—cataracts, glaucoma, depression—are not complications of diabetes, but occur more frequently in people with diabetes and have significant impact upon quality of life for the patient and family.

2 Cataracts

  A Individuals with diabetes are more likely to develop cataracts than individuals without diabetes.

  B Increased polyol pathway activity, due to hyperglycemia, may contribute to lens opacity.

  C Improved blood glucose control is associated with decreased incidence of cataracts.

  D Routine annual eye exams (dilated) are the most effective preventative for vision loss from cataracts.

3 Glaucoma

  A Glaucoma is more common in individuals with diabetes than in individuals without diabetes.

  B There is a linear relationship between the incidence of glaucoma and age, with the incidence increasing with age.

  C The duration of diabetes is related in a linear fashion to an increase in glaucoma.

  D The pathogenesis of the glaucoma in individuals with diabetes is poorly understood at this time.

  E Routine annual eye exams (dilated) are the most effective preventative for vision loss from glaucoma.

4 Depression

  A Depression is not a complication of diabetes but is often a consequence of the complications of diabetes or chronic illness.

  B Depression has a reported incidence of 30% to 70% in patients with diabetes and may be as high as 75% in patients with more than one complication.[46]

  C Assessment for depression among patients with complications is an important role for diabetes educators at all phases in the course of the complication (see Chapter 2, Psychosocial Assessment, in Diabetes Education and Program Management, for more information).

Key Educational Considerations

1 Certain modifiable risk factors (hyperglycemia, hypertension, hyperlipidemia, smoking) play a role in the development of most complications of diabetes.

2 Teach all patients about the benefits of improving blood glucose control since this intervention can be expected to reduce the risks for cardiovascular complications, neuropathy, nephropathy, retinopathy, and cataracts. It also favorably affects lipid levels and platelet adherence.

3 Hypertension is second only to hyperglycemia as a risk factor for the development and progression of diabetic complications. Inform patients that normalization of blood pressure can be expected to reduce the risks for cardiovascular complications, neuropathy, nephropathy, and retinopathy.

4 Treatment of hypertension using an angiotensin-converting enzyme (ACE) inhibitor may be particularly advantageous, unless contraindicated.

5 Medical nutrition therapy and exercise offer direct as well as indirect benefits in reducing the risk for certain complications.

6 Smoking cessation may be especially difficult for patients to accomplish. Assessment of readiness to quit, referral to smoking cessation programs or support groups, alternative nicotine delivery systems, or other cessation aids or medications can be offered at the appropriate time to assist patients in their efforts to quit.

7 Teaching patients behavioral strategies, goal-setting, and problem-solving skills can be useful as they choose and make changes that affect lifestyle-related risk factors.

8 Remembering the modifiable risk factors for diabetes management can be as easy as remembering the motto: "Have good 'CENSE' about diabetes":
Control your glucose, blood pressure, and cholesterol
Early treatment of foot, eye, kidney, and heart problems
No
Smoking
Education about diabetes, nutrition, and exercise

References

1 The DCCT Research Group. The effect of intensive treatment of diabetes on the development and progression of long-term complications in insulin-dependent diabetes mellitus. N Engl J Med. 1993;329:977-86.

2 UK Prospective Diabetes Study Group. Intensive blood-glucose control with sulphonylureas or insulin compared with conventional treatment and risk of complications in patients with type 2 diabetes (UKPD 33). Lancet. 1998;352:837-53.

3 American Diabetes Association. Direct and indirect costs of diabetes in the United States in 1992. Alexandria, Va: 1993.

4 American Diabetes Association. Standards of medical care for patients with diabetes mellitus (position statement). Diabetes Care. 2002;25(suppl 1):S33-S49.

5 American Association of Clinical Endocrinologists. ACE consensus conference on guidelines for glycemic control on the Internet. Available at: http://www.aacecom/pub/press/releases/diabetesconsensuswhitepaper.php. Accessed January 2002.

6 Tull ES, Roseman JM. Diabetes in African Americans. In: National Diabetes Data Group, eds. Diabetes in America. 2nd ed. Bethesda, Md: National Institute of Diabetes and Digestive and Kidney Diseases; 1995. NIH publication 95-1468:613-30.

7 Stern MP, Mitchell BD. Diabetes in Hispanic Americans. In: National Diabetes Data Group, eds. Diabetes in America. 2nd ed. Bethesda, Md: National Institute of Diabetes and Digestive and Kidney Diseases; 1995. NIH publication 95-1468:631-60.

8 Kuhn F, Rackley C. Coronary artery disease in women: risk factors, evaluation, treatment, and prevention. Arch Intern Med. 1993;143:2626-2636.

9 Kuusisto J, Mykkanen L, Pyorala K, Laakso M. NIDDM and its metabolic control predict coronary heart disease in elderly subjects. Diabetes. 1994;43:960-967.

10 UKPDS Group: Tight blood pressure control and risk of macrovascular and microvascular complications in type 2 diabetes (UKPDS 38). BMJ. 1998;317:703-713.

11 American Diabetes Association. Management of dyslipidemia in adults with diabetes (position statement). Diabetes Care 2001;24(suppl 1):S58-S61.

12 Home PD. Insulin resistance is not central to the burden of diabetes. Diabetes Metab Rev. 1997;13:87-92.

13 Colwell JA. Pathophysiology of vascular disease in diabetes: effects of gliclazide. Am J Med. 1991;90(6A):50S-54S.

14 American Diabetes Association. Smoking and diabetes (position statement). Diabetes Care. 2001;24(suppl 1):S64-S65.

15 Haire-Joshu D, Glasgow RE, Tibbs TL. Smoking and diabetes (technical review). Diabetes Care. 1999;22:1887-1898.

16 American Diabetes Association. Nutrition recommendations and principles for people with diabetes (position statement). Diabetes Care. 2002;25(suppl 1):S61-S63.

17 Mayer-Davis EJ, Levin S, Marshall JA. Heterogeneity in associations between macronutrient intake and lipoprotein profile in individuals with type 2 diabetes. Diabetes Care. 1999;22:1632-1639.

18 Manilow MR, Bostom AG, Krauss RM. Homocysteine, diet and cardiovascular disease. A statement for healthcare professionals from the nutrition committee, American Heart Association. Circulation. 1999;99:178-182.

19 Paffenberger RS Jr, Hyde RT, Wing AL, Hsieh CC. Physical activity, all-cause mortality and longevity of college alumni. N Engl J Med. 1986;314:605-613.

20 Lee CD, Blair SN, Jackson AS. Cardiorespiratory fitness, body composition, and all-cause and cardiovascular disease mortality in men. Am J Clin Nutr. 1999;69:373-380.

21 Williams RB Jr, Haney TL, Lee KL, et al. Type A behavior, hostility, and coronary atherosclerosis. Psychosom Med. 1980;42:539-549.

22 Barzilay J, Warram JH, Rand LI, Pfeifer MA, Krolewski AS. Risk for cardiovascular autonomic neuropathy is associated with the HLA-DR3/4 phenotype in type I diabetes mellitus. Ann Intern Med. 1992;116:544-549.

23 Harris M, Eastman R, Cowie C. Symptoms of sensory neuropathy in adults with NIDDM in the US population. Diabetes Care. 1993;16:1446-1452.

24 Sands ML, Shetterly SM, Franklin GM, Hamman RF. Incidence of distal symmetric sensory neuropathy in NIDDM. Diabetes Care. 1997;20:322-329.

25 Gadia MT, Natori N, Ramos LB, Ayyar DR, Skyler JS, Sosenko JM. Influence of height on quantitative sensory, nerve-conduction, and clinical indices of diabetic peripheral neuropathy. Diabetes Care. 1987;10:613-616.

26 Perkins BA, Greene DA, Bril V. Glycemic control is related to the morphological severity of diabetic sensorimotor polyneuropathy. Diabetes Care. 2001;24:748-751.

27 Vinik AI, Milicevic Z, Pittenger GL. Beyond glycemia. Diabetes Care. 1995;18:1037-1041.

28 Reja A, Tesfaye S, Harris ND, Ward JD. Is ACE inhibition with lisinopril helpful in diabetic neuropathy? Diabetic Med. 1995;12:307-309.

29 Adler AI, Boyko EJ, Ahroni JH, et al. Risk factors for diabetic peripheral sensory neuropathy. Results of the Seattle Prospective Diabetes Foot Study. Diabetes Care. 1997;20:1162-1167.

30 Tanenberg RJ, Schumer MP, Greene DA, Pfeifer MA. Neuropathic problems of the lower extremities on diabetic patients. In: Levin and O'Neal's The Diabetic Foot. 6th ed. Bowker JH, Pfeifer MA, eds. St. Louis: Mosby; 2001:33-64.

31 Mayer JH, Tomlinson DR. Prevention of defects of axonal transport and nerve conduction velocity by oral administration of myoinositol or an aldose reductase inhibitor in streptozotocin-diabetic rats. Diabetologia. 1983;25:433-438.

32 Mitchell BD, Hawthorne BD, Hawthorne VM, Vinik AI. Cigarette smoking and neuropathy in diabetic patients. Diabetes Care. 1990;13:434-437.

33 Gohdes D. Diabetes in North American Indians and Alaska Natives. In: National Diabetes Data Group, eds. Diabetes in America. 2nd ed. Bethesda, Md: National Institute of Diabetes and Digestive and Kidney Diseases; 1995, NIH publication 95-1468:683-702.

34 Krolewski AS, Canessa M, Warram JH, et al. Predisposition to hypertension and susceptibility to renal disease in insulin dependent diabetes mellitus. N Engl J Med. 1988;318:140-45.

35 The Microalbumin Captopril Study Group. Captopril reduces the risk of nephropathy in IDDM patients with microalbuminuria. Diabetologia. 1996;39:587-593.

36 Mulec H, Johnson S-A, Björck S. Relationship between serum cholesterol and diabetic nephropathy. Lancet. 1990;335:1537-1538.

37 Tonolo G, Ciccarese M, Brizzi P, et al. Reduction of albumin excretion rate in normotensive microalbuminuric type 2 diabetic patients during long-term simvastatin treatment. Diabetes Care. 1997;20:1891-1895.

38 Franz MJ. Protein controversies in diabetes. Diabetes Spectrum. 2000;13:132-141.

39 Zeller K, Whittaker E, Sullivan L, Raskin P, Jacobson HR. Effect of restricting dietary protein on the progression of renal failure in patients with insulin-dependent diabetes mellitus. N Engl J Med. 1991;324:78-84.

40 Sawicki PT, Didjurgeit U, Mühlhauser I, Bender R, Heinemann L, Berger M. Smoking is associated with progression of diabetic nephropathy. Diabetes Care. 1994;17:126-131.

41 American Diabetes Association. Diabetes mellitus and exercise (position statement). Diabetes Care. 2001;24(suppl 1):S51-S55.

42 Klein R, Klein BEK. Vision disorders in diabetes. In: National Diabetes Data Group, eds. Diabetes in America. 2nd ed. Bethesda, Md: National Institute of Diabetes and Digestive and Kidney Diseases, 1995;293-338.

43 American Diabetes Association. Diabetic retinopathy (position statement). Diabetes Care. 2001;24(suppl l):S73-S76.

44 Rand LI, Krolewski AS, Aiello LM, Warram JH, Baker RS, Maki T. Multiple factors in the prediction of risk of proliferative diabetic retinopathy. N Engl J Med. 1985;113:1433-1438.

45 Chaturvedi N, Sjolie AK, Stephenson JM, et al. Effect of lisinopril on progression of retinopathy in normotensive people with type 1 diabetes. The EUCLID study group. EURODIAB controlled trial of lisinopril in insulin-dependent diabetes mellitus. Lancet. 1998;351:28-31.

46 Goodnick PJ, Henry JH, Buki VM. Treatment of depression in patients with diabetes mellitus. J Clin Psychiatry. 1995;56(4)128-136.

Suggested Readings

American Diabetes Association: Clinical Practice Recommendations 2001. Diabetes Care. 2001;24 (supplement 1).

Bowker J, Pfeifer MA, eds. The Diabetic Foot. 6th ed. Philadelphia: Mosby; 2001.

Cavallerano JD. Protect your vision. Diabetes Forecast. Sept 1999:53-57.

Chantrel F, Moulin B, Hannedouche T. Blood pressure, diabetes and diabetic nephropathy. Diabetes & Metabolism. 2000;26(4):37-44.

Clark CM, Lee, DA. Prevention and treatment of the complications of diabetes mellitus. N Engl J Med. 1995;332:1210-1217.

D'Arrigo, T. Women, type 2 and cardiovascular risk. Diabetes Forecast. 1999;Jan:31-33.

Dinsmoor RS. AGE's—closing in on complications. Diabetes Self-Management. 1997;14(2):6-10.

Eastman RC, Javitt JC, Herman WH, et al. Model of complications of NIDDM. I. Model construction and assumptions. Diabetes Care. 1997;20:725-734.

Eastman RC, Javitt JC, Herman WH, et al. Model of complications of NIDDM. II Analysis of the health benefits and cost-effectiveness of treating NIDDM with the goal of normoglycemia. Diabetes Care. 1997;20:735-737.

Estacio RO, Jeffers BW, Gifford N, Schrier RW. Effect of blood pressure control on diabetic microvascular complications in patients with hypertension and type 2 diabetes. Diabetes Care. 2000;23(suppl 2):54-64.

Greene DA, Feldman EL, Stevens MJ, Sima AAF, Albers JW, Pfeifer MA. Diabetic neuropathy. In: Porte Jr D, Sherwin RS, eds. Ellenberg and Rifkin's Diabetes Mellitus. 5th ed. New York: Elsevier Science Publishing; 1997:1009-1076.

Hinson J, Riordan K, Hemphill O, Randolph C, Fonesca V. Hypertension education: an important and neglected part of the diabetes education curriculum. The Diabetes Educ. 1997;23:166-170.

Klein, R. Hyperglycemia and microvascular and macrovascular disease in diabetes. Diabetes Care. 1995;18:258-268.

LeMone P. The physical effects of diabetes on sexuality in women. The Diabetes Educ. 1996;22:361-366.

Levine ME, Pfeifer MA. The Uncomplicated Guide to Diabetes Complications. Alexandria, Va: American Diabetes Association; 1997.

Low P, Panel Members of the American Academy of Neurology. Assessment. Clinical autonomic testing report of the therapeutics and technology assessment subcommittee of the American Academy of Neurology. Neurology. 1996;46:873-880.

Marks JB, Raskin P. Cardiovascular risk in diabetes: a brief review. Journal of Diabetes & its Complications. 2000;14:108-115.

Reno PL, Arfken CL, Herns JM, Fisher EB. Factors that influence the decision to receive treatment for proliferative diabetic retinopathy. The Diabetes Educ. 1997;23: 653-655.

Rovner JF. Diabetes and the brain: a complex relationship. Diabetes Spectrum. 1997;10: 23-70.

Spollett GR. Assessment and management of erectile dysfunction in men with diabetes. The Diabetes Educ. 1999;25:65-73.

Walker EA, Wylie-Rosett J, Shamoon H, et al. Program development to prevent complications of diabetes: assessment of barriers in an urban clinic. Diabetes Care. 1995;18:1291-1293.

Wannamethee SG, Shaper AG, Alberti KG. Physical activity, metabolic factors, and the incidence of coronary heart disease and type 2 diabetes. Arch Intern Med. 2000;160: 2108-2116.

Learning Assessment: Post-Test Questions

Chronic Complications of Diabetes: An Overview   3

1 Risk factors (choose one):
  A Are unique to persons with diabetes and are a significant predictor of the progression of the disease
  B Can be attributed to a single etiology and are important to the development of diabetic complications
  C May vary for each complication contributing to a highly variable, individual, and complex pattern of disease progression
  D Affect individuals with diabetes similarly at approximately similar ages and stages of diabetes pathogenesis

2 Which of the following statements best describes the role of hyperglycemia in the development of complications of diabetes?
  A There is strong evidence that control of hyperglycemia will result in a decrease in cardiovascular events
  B Improved glycemic control has a marginal impact, if any, on the total cholesterol levels, platelet adherence factors, and LDL cholesterol
  C Elevated blood glucose levels can interfere with nerve membrane functioning and nerve transport
  D Hyperglycemia leads to suppression of the polyol pathway and the formation of advanced glycation end products (AGE)

3 When compared to Caucasians with diabetes, African Americans with diabetes have a lower overall prevalence rate for:
  A Myocardial infarction
  B Hypertension
  C Neuropathy
  D Nephropathy

4 In addition to the nonmodifiable risk factors of duration of diabetes, race, genetics, and age, for which of the following complications of diabetes has height and autoimmunity been shown to be a factor?
  A Cardiovascular complications
  B Neuropathies
  C Nephropathies
  D Retinopathies

5 Angiotensin-converting enzyme inhibitor (ACE-I) can slow the progression of which of the following complications of diabetes?
  A Retinopathies
  B Neuropathies
  C Nephropathies
  D All of the above

6 Which of the following supplements appear to help maintain nerve function?
  A Chromium and St. John's Wort
  B Myoinositol and gamma-linoleic acid (GLA)
  C Chromium and GLA
  D Vitamin B_2 and myoinositol

7 Which of the following is the most costly complication of diabetes?
  A Retinopathy
  B Cardiovascular disease
  C Nephropathy
  D Neuropathy

8 Which of the following increase the risk of diabetic nephropathy?
  A Hyperglycemia
  B Hypertension
  C Hypercholesterolemia
  D All of the above

9 The need for laser therapy for diabetic retinopathy has only a small increase after how many years duration of diabetes?
  A 5 years
  B 10 years
  C 17 years
  D 22 years

10 Which of the following is more common in people with diabetes?
  A Cataracts
  B Retinopathy
  C Glaucoma
  D All of the above

See next page for answer key.

Post-Test Answer Key

Chronic Complications of Diabetes: An Overview 3

1 C

2 C

3 A

4 B

5 D

6 B

7 C

8 D

9 D

10 D

A Core Curriculum for Diabetes Education
Diabetes and Complications

Diabetic Foot Care and Education 4

Jessie H. Ahroni, PhD, ARNP, CDE
Veterans Affairs Puget Sound Health Care System
School of Nursing, University of Washington
Seattle, Washington

Introduction

1 Teaching patients and healthcare professionals how to reduce the risk factors for lower-extremity complications is an important strategy in diabetes management.

2 Appropriate diabetes self-management education and preventive foot care are known to reduce lower-extremity complications. This knowledge must be transferred to patients with diabetes, since they are the only ones who can translate this information into self-care behaviors.

Objectives

Upon completion of this chapter, the learner will be able to
1 Identify the effects of peripheral sensory neuropathy, autonomic neuropathy, and motor neuropathy on the functions of the foot.
2 Identify the signs of peripheral vascular disease in the lower extremities of people with diabetes.
3 List the basic elements of a diabetic foot screening examination.
4 Explain what findings from a foot examination would cause a person with diabetes to be classified as high risk.
5 Describe treatment plans for a person with high-risk feet or a foot ulcer.
6 List guidelines for teaching foot care to both low-risk and high-risk individuals.

Lower-Extremity Complications

1 Diabetic foot complications are costly, but beyond the financial concerns are the inevitable social and psychological distresses to patients and their families.

2 Despite many major advances in healthcare delivery over the last decade, foot problems continue to exact a heavy toll on the quality of life of people with diabetes.[1-5]

3 Amputation is one of the most feared and disabling consequences of long-term uncontrolled diabetes.

4 Certain ethnic groups may be at risk for diabetes-related lower-extremity amputations.
   A Amputation rates based on hospital discharges are generally higher for African Americans than for Caucasians after adjusting for age.[6]
   B For Native Americans living on the Gila River Indian Reservation, the incidence of amputations was 24.1 per 1000 patient years compared with 6.5 per 1000 patient years for the general US diabetic population.[7]
   C Others have reported estimated age-adjusted diabetic amputation rates to be higher in African Americans than in Hispanics or non-Hispanic whites, although Hispanics had a higher proportion of amputations associated with diabetes than African Americans.[8]
   D Population-based data seldom contain the information necessary to control for the potential confounding effects of socioeconomic status and access to health care. Selby and Zhang found that African Americans did not have an increased risk for diabetes-related amputation when access to medical care was comparable.[9]

5 The prognosis of people with diabetes who have undergone an amputation is poor.

A In one study, the 2-year survival rate after a diabetes-related amputation was 50%. Five-year mortality following amputation ranged from 39% to 68%.[10]

B The chance of a new or second leg amputation within 1 year of the first amputation has been estimated at 9% to 20%.[10] Within 5 years of an initial amputation, 28% to 51% of surviving amputees with diabetes have undergone a second leg amputation.[11]

C Survivors of amputation report a lower quality of life and often are not successfully rehabilitated into the community.[12]

6 Lower-extremity complications are a significant cause of hospitalization, disability, morbidity, and mortality among people with diabetes. Improvements in the prevention of diabetes-related foot ulceration and amputation are needed to avoid their considerable medical, social, and economic costs.

A In a 1986 cost-of-illness study assessing the economic costs of type 2 diabetes in the United States, chronic skin ulcers alone were estimated to account for $250 million in healthcare expenditures.[13]

B Approximately $500 million was spent in the United States in 1988 for the care of people with diabetes and foot problems.[11]

C A more recent economic study in Sweden estimated the 1995 value cost per patient in US dollars for diabetes-related foot complications.[14]

- For patients with ischemia who healed, the estimated cost was $26 700 US dollars.
- For patients without ischemia who healed, the estimated cost was $16 100 US dollars.
- For patients with an amputation who healed, the corresponding costs were $43 100 US dollars after a minor (below ankle) amputation and $63 100 US dollars after a major (above ankle) amputation.

D The number of hospital discharges listing an amputation and diabetes in the National Hospital Discharge Survey was 67 000 in 1994.[15] This number underestimates the problem because diabetes is not listed on the discharge record for 40% of all hospitalizations of people with diabetes.[16,17]

E Lower-extremity complications of diabetes result from a combination of contributing causes rather than from a single cause. The pathophysiological factors that lead to diabetic foot complications are neuropathy, ischemia, trauma, ulceration, faulty wound healing, infection, and gangrene.[18]

Neuropathies

1 Sensory, autonomic, and motor neuropathies act synergistically to cause diabetic foot complications.

2 Peripheral sensory polyneuropathy is a major pathophysiologic risk factor for foot ulceration and amputation.

A About 50% of people with diabetes of 15 years' duration have peripheral sensory neuropathy.[17] Loss of protective sensation allows trauma to go undetected by the patient.

B The earliest and most severe damage due to diffuse, somatic, bilateral, distal symmetrical polyneuropathy occurs at the most distal enervated sites in a "stocking and glove" distribution.[19] Loss of protective sensation affects the toes and feet first, although sensorimotor functions of the fingers and hands may also be impaired.

C A quick and easy way to identify feet without protective sensation is to evaluate the ability of the patient to perceive the pressure of a 5.07 monofilament applied to the most common sites of potential ulceration. These sites are the plantar surface of the great toe and fifth toe, the plantar metatarsal heads (first and fifth), and the heel (see Figure 4.1).

Figure 4.1. Sites for Monofilament Assessment

Suggested sites on the feet to test for protective sensation using a 5.07 monofilament.

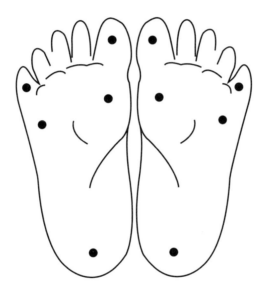

- A 5.07 monofilament delivers 10 g of linear pressure when it is bent into a "C" shape. Inability to perceive the monofilament at any site is evidence of neuropathy.[20]
- Educators and providers who wish to use this tool should obtain instructions and practice under supervision before incorporating this test into their practice.
- This procedure should be demonstrated first in an area of intact sensation, such as on the arm.
- The examiner should then use the modified, 2-alternative, forced-choice method to test the most common sites of potential ulceration.[20]
- Sensory neuropathy is diagnosed if the 5.07 monofilament cannot be perceived at any site on either foot.
- The 5.07 monofilament is the single most practical tool for discriminating between those with protective sensation and those without it.[21]

3 Autonomic neuropathy causes changes in the nerves that control blood flow, perspiration, skin hydration, and possibly bone composition of the foot.[22]

A Lack of adequate skin hydration leads to dry skin, which can result in cracking and fissures of the skin on the foot. Dry, cracked skin can be a portal for the microorganisms that cause infection. Areas of callus are particularly prone to dryness.

B There may be changes in blood flow due to autonomic neuropathy that result in vasodilatation and shunting of blood away from the nutrient capillary bed.[23]

C Autonomic neuropathy may impair the body's ability to mount an inflammatory response to trauma and infection in diabetic feet. This lack of an inflammatory response may contribute to skin ischemia and faulty wound healing and an impaired ability to fight infection.[24]

D Some experts propose that vasodilatation and shunting of blood flow may cause bone demineralization and osteolysis that contribute to changes in the shape of the foot.[22] Charcot's foot is an extreme example of such changes.
  • In the acute stage of Charcot's foot, the foot becomes warm, swollen, and erythematous; this condition may be difficult to differentiate from infection.
  • Although patients with Charcot's foot changes generally have severe sensory neuropathy, they also may experience pain or tenderness. Because of relative insensitivity, however, many patients continue to walk, which creates stress fractures and further disruption of the joint architecture.
  • The changes of Charcot's foot may occur in the forefoot, midfoot, or hindfoot, although the most common presentation is collapse of the longitudinal arch. Diabetes educators should refer all patients suspected of having an acute Charcot's foot or a sudden change in foot shape for orthopedic evaluation.
  • Aggressive treatment in the early stage of Charcot's foot focuses on stabilizing the foot in a functional position, usually with a total contact cast. Without this treatment, the foot may develop a "rocker bottom" configuration or other bony prominence on the plantar surface that is prone to ulceration.[25] Once the Charcot's foot stabilizes, protective shoes to accommodate the changes in foot shape may be needed to prevent ulceration.

4 Motor neuropathy leads to muscle atrophy that results in weakness and changes in foot shape.

  A Weak intrinsic muscles allow flexors to predominate. The diabetic foot may take on a pes cavus shape, with a high arch and prominent metatarsal heads. The fat pad that normally protects the metatarsal heads at the ball of the foot becomes displaced.

  B Dominant flexors also cause the toes to become deformed in a hammer or claw shape. Such muscle imbalances and abnormalities lead to irregular weight bearing and areas of high plantar pressure.

  C There may also be subtle changes in posture and gait that cause changes in weight bearing and plantar pressure.[26]

  D Assessment that reveals muscle atrophy or changes in foot shape necessitates further orthopedic evaluation and shoes that are constructed to accommodate foot changes and alleviate points of excess pressure.

5 Peripheral vascular disease causes an inadequate blood supply (ischemia) to the lower limbs, which deprives the tissues of oxygen and nutrients and impairs the removal of waste products.

  A Ischemia results primarily from atherosclerosis, which occurs early in the course of diabetes and progresses rapidly. Atherosclerosis is associated with other risk factors such as aging, male gender, dyslipidemia, hypertension, smoking, obesity, a sedentary lifestyle, hyperglycemia, and hyperinsulinemia.[27] Thrombi from infection or blood clots can also cause ischemic changes.

B People with diabetes are more likely to have vascular disease below the knee. The estimated prevalence of arteriosclerosis obliterans, which totally occludes a vessel, is 15% after a 10-year duration of diabetes and 45% after 20 years.[28]

C Symptoms of peripheral vascular disease include intermittent claudication, cold feet, and pain at rest that is relieved by dependency.

D Vascular bypass surgery or angioplasty may enhance blood flow and improve the wound-healing process. However, arteriosclerosis is present not only in the larger vessels treated by these methods but also in the tiny vessels that supply blood to the skin. These smaller vessels are not amenable to surgical interventions.

E The single most important treatment for peripheral vascular disease is smoking cessation.[29] Self-management education should include risks faced by patients with diabetes who smoke, smoking cessation strategies, alternative nicotine devices, and referrals to aid in stopping smoking.

Edema

1 Edema, whether from local infection or systemic causes, can adversely affect skin texture, cutaneous circulation, and wound healing.[30] When edema is present, it is wise to have the patient examined by a clinician to determine the cause of the edema.

A If edema is due to venous insufficiency alone, then compression hose, which can be obtained from a well-stocked pharmacy, drugstore, or medical supply store, may be useful. The patient's legs should be carefully measured as described on the packaging and the stockings fitted so as not to restrict arterial flow.

B If there is arterial insufficiency, compression hose may be contraindicated or the amount of compression may need to be reduced.

C Elevating the extremity above the heart may control dependent edema, but diuretics may be required for some patients.

D If edema is due to congestive heart failure, it may indicate a need for a change in medication. In the case of heart failure, reducing edema by leg elevation or compression may increase the fluid return and could potentially lead to volume overload.

E When arterial flow is severely compromised, patients may not be able to tolerate leg elevation and may even need to sit with the feet dependent to facilitate blood flow to the feet.

Trauma

1 A 1990 study of 80 amputations revealed that in 69 of the cases, the initial precipitating event was preventable minor trauma leading to skin ulceration.[18] Common sources of trauma include poorly fitting shoes, ingrown toenails, wrinkled stockings, foreign objects in the shoe, walking barefoot or sock footed, and inappropriate care of toenails, corns, and calluses.

2 Chemical trauma results when caustic substances such as over-the-counter corn and callus removers destroy fragile tissue.

3 Thermal injuries can occur from hot foot soaks, hot water bottles, heating pads, or walking on hot sand and pavement, resulting in severe burns to the insensate and vascularly compromised foot.

   A In a diabetic foot affected by autonomic neuropathy, the foot may become continually vasodilated.

   B Applying heat to a diabetic foot increases metabolic demands. Tissue damage may occur when the vascular system is unable to meet the increased metabolic demands or unable to further vasodilate or sweat to release heat because of autonomic neuropathy.

4 Most skin ulcers are caused by minor, repetitive pressure with each step (eg, walking on a bony, plantar prominence in a shoe with insufficient insole and sole cushioning) rather than a single episode of identifiable trauma.[31]

5 Most amputations resulting from trauma can be prevented through patient education and effective self-care that emphasizes properly fitting protective footwear.

Ulceration

1 A *foot ulceration* is a full-thickness skin defect below the malleoli that penetrates to the subcutaneous tissue.[32]

2 Any wound on the foot of a person with diabetes is a cause for serious concern regardless of the depth or size.

3 Diabetic foot ulceration need not result in infection or amputation. Proper wound management can heal many foot ulcers, and most amputations are preventable.

   A There is disagreement on the details of foot ulcer management for people with diabetes; however, there is substantial agreement on the major principles of such care:[33]
   - Optimizing glycemic control, nutrition, and hydration
   - Controlling sepsis
   - Debriding necrotic tissues
   - Applying dressings
   - Treating local edema
   - Requiring bed rest or limited ambulation
   - Utilizing protective footwear to redistribute weight and relieve pressure
   - Providing foot care self-management education

Infection

1 The presence of purulence (pus), significant erythema, increased local warmth, tenderness, induration, fluctuance, or drainage indicates infection. If a diabetic foot lesion is infected, appropriate oral or parenteral antimicrobial therapy is prescribed after cultures are obtained, preferably by deep-tissue curettage.[34]

2 Acute or subacute infection (of less than 30 days' duration) without systemic symptoms, gangrene, or osteomyelitis can effectively be treated using a single oral antibiotic for 2 weeks, with frequent follow-up and daily wound care.[34]

A Gram-positive aerobic organisms, particularly staphylococci and streptococci, cause most foot infections in people with diabetes.

B Initial antibiotic therapy must cover these organisms and can be extended according to culture results or lack of clinical response.[34]

3 Patients with fever, leukocytosis, severe hyperglycemia, acidosis, hypotension, extensive cellulitis, lymphangitis, deep space infections, gangrene, crepitus, gas in the tissues, evidence of osteomyelitis, or failure of previous courses of therapy need to be admitted to the hospital for parenteral antibiotics and surgical drainage if necessary.[34] Patients who cannot perform or obtain needed outpatient care are also candidates for hospitalization.

Gangrene

1 *Gangrene* is a nonspecific term for tissue death. Microthrombi that develop as a result of infection, arteriosclerosis, or other decreased blood flow, vasculitis, or increased platelet aggregation can cause a complete blockage of the delivery of oxygen and nutrients to the tissue, resulting in tissue death or necrosis.

2 Dry gangrene is associated with ischemia. When the gangrenous portion is sharply demarcated and affects only a small area, it may be left untreated but closely observed. In some cases, the affected part, usually a toe tip, will mummify and auto-amputate.

3 A wet or moist gangrenous area is a sign that the process of tissue death is progressive or that infection may be involved. Because of the complete blockage of blood flow to the necrotic area, surgical intervention is usually required.

Identifying the Foot at Risk

1 Identification of the foot at risk for diabetic complications can be done through screening of people who are asymptomatic.

A Screening allows classification regarding the likelihood of having a particular disease or outcome.

B *Screening* is a test, procedure, or examination that does not diagnose but simply identifies those who are at high risk.

2 A study at the Veterans Affairs Puget Sound Health Care System, Seattle Division, used 2 stepwise logistic regression models to identify risk factors to predict diabetic foot ulceration and amputation.[35]

A The variables that predicted foot ulceration were
- Sensory neuropathy (inability to perceive a 5.07 monofilament)
- History of amputation
- Absent toe vibration (using a 128-cycle tuning fork)
- Insulin treatment
- History of ulceration

B When none of the 5 variables were present, the probability of foot ulceration was 0.05%. When all 5 variables were present, the probability of foot ulceration was

68% and the likelihood ratio was 11 times. The likelihood ratio summarizes the odds of foot ulceration after a positive screening test.

C The 5 variables that predicted amputation were
- History of foot ulceration or amputation
- Charcot's foot deformity
- Diabetes duration greater than 10 years
- Hammer or claw toes
- Self-reported nephropathy

D When none of the 5 variables were present, the probability of an amputation was 0.05%. When all 5 variables were present, the probability of an amputation was 84% and the likelihood ratio was 164 times. The likelihood ratio summarizes the odds of amputation after a positive screening test.

E The presence of 3 of the multivariate criteria for predicting foot ulceration (history of ulceration, history of amputation, and insulin treatment), and possibly all 5 of the criteria for amputation, can be detected by asking the patient questions. Those who have had a foot ulceration or amputation can automatically be categorized as high risk; no further screening questions or examinations are necessary to make this determination.

3 A foot examination is a powerful way to teach the importance of foot care. A thorough foot examination should be performed at least once a year, and patients should be asked about foot problems at every visit. A standardized assessment form that lists the specific screening activities that need to be done, the interventions recommended, and foot-risk categories can be used to document the examination.[36] By taking advantage of this time the educator can emphasize the importance of this self-care activity and use the opportunity for individualized instruction.

A A *foot-risk screening* involves assessing changes in the feet since the last visit. Areas to address include a history of peripheral vascular disease, intermittent claudication, symptoms of neuropathy, and a history of foot ulceration or amputation.

B Record the presence or absence of current foot ulceration. If ulceration is present, refer the patient to a provider with expertise in foot care or to a wound care clinic for ongoing care.

C A vision assessment using a handheld or wall-mounted Snellen chart can help determine whether patients can see their feet well enough to perform an accurate visual inspection.
- Vision that is regarded as mildly to moderately impaired is probably inadequate for performing a reliable foot inspection.
- If vision is poor, a manual inspection may substitute for the visual inspection.
- If impaired mobility makes it difficult for patients to reach their feet, a mirror, magnifying glass, or magnifying mirror may be used if vision is adequate.
- When both vision and mobility are impaired, a family member or other caregiver may need to assist with daily foot inspection.

D In the clinical setting, sensory examination with a 5.07 monofilament is the single most practical measure for detecting neuropathy.

E Daily visual or manual foot inspection is recommended for patients with neuropathy.
- A foot inspection consists of a brief examination of color, skin integrity, and toenail length in good light, such as when drying off after a shower or bath or when putting on socks. Areas to inspect include the tops, bottoms, and sides of each

foot and between the toes. Ask patients to demonstrate their ability to reach the feet for foot care and manual inspection.

- Although patients without neuropathy are likely to be able to perceive injuries to their feet, daily foot inspection is a good habit for all people with diabetes to develop to promote early problem recognition and intervention.

4 The probability of vascular disease can be determined from knowledge of the patient's age, history of vascular disease, venous filling time, and examination of the lower-extremity pulses by palpation.[37] Segmental Doppler blood pressures and calculation of the ankle-arm index (AAI) need not be performed to determine the risk for diabetic foot complications.

A Palpation of the dorsalis pedis (DP) and posterior tibialis (PT) pulses should be performed and recorded as either present or absent.

B The AAI should be determined in patients without palpable pulses or those otherwise suspected of having vascular disease of the lower extremities.

C Venous filling time is easily determined.

- After identifying a prominent pedal vein, the examiner assists the patient in elevating the legs to a 45° angle for 1 minute.
- The patient is then asked to sit up and hang the legs over the side of the examining table.
- The time in seconds until the veins bulge above the skin level is recorded.
- The time to reappearance of the veins can be recorded or results can be classified as normal (≤20 seconds) or abnormal (>20 seconds).
- Those patients with ischemia who would benefit from vascular bypass surgery or angioplasty should be referred to appropriate healthcare providers.

5 Structural deformities are identified during the physical examination. The presence or absence of prominent metatarsal heads, hammer or claw toes, Charcot's foot deformity (collapse of the foot arch), bony prominences (exostosis), hallux valgus (bunion), or hallux limitus (also called hallux rigidus, stiff great toe joint with limited range of motion), and corns and calluses are recorded.

6 Footwear assessment is another important part of the foot examination. This is an ideal time to inspect the shoes and socks worn by patients and to offer personalized information about footwear.

A Point out the need for shoes with cushioned insoles and soles. Generally shoes made from soft materials are best. They should be constructed with laces or Velcro® closing for adjustability and have seams that do not rub bony prominences.

B If claw or hammer toes are present, advise the patient to wear shoes with plenty of toe room (eg, extra-depth or custom-made footwear).

C People with severe foot deformities need custom footwear that is available by prescription from foot care specialists, pedorthists, orthotists, or podiatrists.

7 Skin abnormalities are also evaluated during the foot examination. Common abnormalities include excessive dryness and macerated, intertrigous areas that indicate severe tinea pedis (athlete's foot fungus).

A Dry skin can be treated with daily emollients or moisturizers. The best time to apply these agents is after a bath or shower. Emollients and moisturizers should not be applied between the toes.

B Soaking the feet is not routinely recommended for people with diabetes. In addition to the risk of hot water burns, soaking removes the natural skin oils and can open small cracks in the skin, creating a portal for bacteria. Repeatedly wetting and drying the feet can worsen dry skin problems.

C Tinea pedis can be treated with increased attention to drying between the toes and using over-the-counter antifungal agents. Some patients find that loosely lacing pieces of lamb's wool between the toes helps prevent maceration and fungal infections. Fungal infections that are severe or persistent should be brought to the attention of a medical provider.

D Corns and calloused areas are signs of increased pressure.
  • Excess keratin may be gently filed or buffed with an emery board or pumice stone.
  • Over-the-counter corn and callus removers may cause burns or ulcers. Extremely thick corns or calluses need to be treated by a foot care specialist.

8 Toenail deformities such as fungal dystrophy (thickened and deformed toenails) or ingrown toenails should be recorded during the foot examination. Fungal toenail infections (tinea unguium, also called onychomycosis) that require treatment should be brought to the attention of the medical provider.

A To properly trim nails, the patient or caregiver should be taught to cut or file the toenails to the contour of the toe, being sure that all sharp edges are filed smoothly.

B If the patient does not see well or has difficulty reaching the feet, a family member, nurse, or podiatrist can help with nail care.

C Patients with extremely thick toenails or ingrown toenails should be referred to a foot care specialist for treatment.

9 Risk determination and planning are done at the end of the foot examination. A foot risk category is determined and reviewed with the patient. A plan should then be made for foot care education and annual foot exams (for low-risk patients). High-risk patients require more frequent foot exams and more detailed, personalized education emphasizing daily inspection, protective footwear, and the need to report foot problems promptly.

How to Teach About Foot Care

1 Before teaching foot care skills, the educator needs to assess the patient's present knowledge, behaviors, beliefs, and abilities by asking "What are you doing now to care for your feet?"

2 The challenge for the educator is to provide information that is tailored to the patient's individual risk level and current foot care practices.

3 Homelessness or blindness are situations for which the educator must adapt instructions to meet these patients' special needs.

4 Patients need to be given practical and realistic information about foot care that is presented in positive statements as "dos" rather than "don'ts." Give reasons why foot care is important and the purpose of recommendations.

5 It is helpful for patients to have some written guidelines about foot care to take home.
  A Give patients only one handout at each visit that emphasizes an important foot care concept, such as
  • A reminder poster to hang on the back of the bathroom door or a large-print or low-literacy version with graphics
  • Reprints of articles written for the lay population

6 To help personalize the information, the educator can highlight sections of an article that emphasizes essential principles and cross out information that is not applicable.

7 Provide materials that are appropriate for the patient's language and literacy level.

What to Teach About Foot Care

1 Teach patients with diabetes the basic principles of foot care. Patients with neuropathy, vascular disease, or a history of foot ulceration or amputation should periodically be assessed for foot care practices and provided with personalized foot care education.

2 For high-risk patients, review the principles of foot care at every visit. For low-risk patients, an annual assessment and review is probably sufficient. Encourage patients to remove their shoes and socks at every healthcare visit, even if they are not asked to do so.

3 Teach and review the following principles of foot care.
  A Look at your feet and interdigital areas daily (eg, whenever putting on or taking off socks). A magnifying glass, mirror, or magnifying mirror may be helpful in examining the top, bottom, and sides of the feet for color and skin integrity.
  • Have the patient perform a return demonstration after explaining and demonstrating a foot inspection. Point out areas that need special attention.
  • If the patient is unable to do a demonstration, a family member or other care provider can perform the inspection.
  B Inspect shoes daily by feeling the inside of the shoe for torn or loose linings, cracks, pebbles, nails, or other loose objects and irregularities that may irritate the skin. Get in the habit of shaking out your shoes before putting them on.
  • Soft leather or canvas shoes that have cushioned insoles and fit well at the time of purchase offer the best protection.
  • Shoes need to match the shape of the foot in both length and width and should be deep enough to accommodate any deformities.
  • Changing shoes during the day can limit repetitive local pressure.
  C Avoid going barefoot or sock footed. Wear footwear at the pool or beach. Use sunscreen to avoid burns.
  D Wash and dry the feet thoroughly, especially between the toes.
  E Use a thin layer of lamb's wool to separate toes that overlap or touch each other and to prevent maceration.
  F Caution patients to avoid burns from hot water by checking the water temperature of the bath or shower with the forearm, elbow, or a bath thermometer.
  G Avoid routine foot soaks.

H Moisturize dry skin (except between the toes) with an emollient such as lanolin or hand lotion. Hand lotions containing alcohol are not suitable because the alcohol may contribute to drying or cracking of the skin.

I Cut toenails straight across and file the sharp corners to match the contour of the toe, making sure that all sharp edges are filed smooth. If the patient does not see well or has difficulty reaching the feet, a family member, nurse, or podiatrist can do this self-care task.

J Avoid self-treatment of corns, calluses, or ingrown toenails.
- Using chemicals, sharp instruments, or razor blades to treat these problems can lead to ulceration or infection.
- A patient or family member may gently buff corns or calluses with an emery board or pumice stone. Emollient lotion or cream should then be applied to keep the corn or callus soft.
- Flaky fungal debris can be loosened and removed with a soft nailbrush during regular bathing.

K Wear well-fitting, soft cotton, synthetic blend, or wool socks. Avoid using hot water bottles, heating pads, or microwave foot warmers because they can cause burns.

L Seek prompt medical attention for any problems (eg, cuts, blisters, calluses, any wounds that do not heal, or signs of infection such as redness, swelling, pus, drainage, or fever).

M Treat fungal infections promptly with antifungal cream, spray, or powder. Change footwear periodically to keep the area between the toes clean and dry. Severe fungal infections should be brought to the attention of the medical provider in case prescription medications are required.

Key Educational Considerations

1 Appropriate diabetes education and preventive care can reduce the risk of foot complications in susceptible patients.

2 Meticulous foot care and proper patient education has been reported to reduce the amputation rate associated with diabetes by 50%.[38]

3 Teaching patients and healthcare professionals ways to reduce risk factors and prevent limb loss due to foot disease is an important strategy in diabetes management and cost reduction.

4 Predicting which patients are at the greatest risk could lead to more efficient use of resources.

5 Because present knowledge regarding the prevention and management of diabetic foot disease is not widely applied in practice, rates of foot ulcers and major amputations in the United States remain high.

6 For people without established end-stage complications of diabetes, better control of blood glucose levels has been shown to reduce the development of neuropathy and slow its progression.

7 According to the strategy of prevention, significantly improving the glycemic control of the entire population of people with diabetes, thus lowering the incidence of risk factors and other complications, is likely to be more effective in preventing foot ulceration and amputation than focusing efforts only on members of the population already at high risk.

Self-Review Questions

1 What steps should be included in every diabetic foot risk screening examination?
2 Describe changes in the appearance of the foot due to autonomic, motor, and sensory neuropathies.
3 List the signs of peripheral vascular disease.
4 Describe the indicators of a high-risk diabetic foot.
5 What is the best test for detecting peripheral sensory neuropathy?
6 Describe 3 preventive measures for diabetic foot problems.
7 State why products for the skin that contain alcohol should be avoided.

Learning Assessment: Case Study 1

WS is an obese 68-year-old man who has had type 2 diabetes for 13 years. He maintains his HbA1c in the target range with NPH and regular insulin twice a day. He is referred to you for foot care education. He does not have a history of peripheral vascular disease, retinopathy, nephropathy, foot ulceration, or amputation. He is insensate to the 5.07 monofilament at several sites on each foot. He has thin, bony feet with a high arch, prominent metatarsal heads, clawed toes, and dry skin. WS is wearing well-worn loafers with no insoles and thin leather soles. He says he is not overly concerned about his feet and tends to only look at them when toweling off after a shower.

Questions for Discussion

1 How would you classify WS' risk for foot ulceration?
2 What aspects of foot care education are important to emphasize for someone at this risk level?
3 What kind of modifications to the general instructions might you anticipate making?

Discussion

1 This patient has neuropathy and is at high risk for foot ulceration or amputation. Being insulin treated and having had diabetes for more than 10 years also increases his risk for diabetic foot complications.

2 Before teaching foot care skills, the educator needs to assess WS' present knowledge, behaviors, beliefs, and abilities.

3 It is essential to assess if WS can see functionally and reach his feet before teaching is begun.
   A Wearing loafers may be a sign that he is unable to bend over to tie shoes.
   B Wearing shirt styles that are easier to put on (eg, pullover versus button) may be a clue to possible neuropathy of the hands.

4 Explain to WS that you are concerned that his casual inspection is no longer adequate because his feet are now insensate. Recommend that he closely examine his feet daily and use a mirror if necessary.

   A Good opportunities to examine the feet are while drying them after bathing, when putting on socks, when getting ready for bed, or when applying emollients to dry skin.

   B Remind him to not put the emollient between his toes. However, he should still examine the areas between the toes.

   C If WS is unable to inspect his feet daily, ask about other family members or caregivers that might be able to assist in performing this inspection.

5 WS's current shoes are not ideal diabetic footwear because of their lack of support, both inside and outside.

   A If he has or can obtain financial resources, athletic shoes with a cushioned sole and insole and a rounded toe box will offer protection.

   B Shoes with Velcro® straps may be easier for him to fasten than those with shoelaces. If this type of shoe is not available commercially, a pedorthotist or cobbler can make this alteration in shoes with laces.

   C Medicare may offer coverage for therapeutic shoes, inserts, and shoe modifications for certain people with diabetes. Information and claim forms can be obtained from the Department of Health and Human Services.

Learning Assessment: Case Study 2

A 20-year-old female (SA) with type 1 diabetes diagnosed 5 years ago has been referred to you for diabetes education. You notice that she has recently started smoking. She is afraid of the complications of diabetes, especially amputation, and intends to do everything possible to prevent these. She does not have any complications of diabetes at this time and can perceive the 5.07 monofilament at all sites tested on each foot. SA's feet are shaped normally and she is wearing high-quality athletic shoes.

Questions for Discussion

1 How would you classify SA's risk for foot ulceration?
2 What aspects of foot care education are important for someone at this risk level?

Discussion

1 SA does not have neuropathy, a history of foot ulceration or amputation, or other complications of diabetes or foot deformities. She currently has a low risk of foot complications.

2 Before teaching foot care skills, the educator needs to assess SA's present knowledge, behaviors, beliefs, and abilities.

3 Although SA has sensation on all parts of her feet, performing a daily foot inspection is a good habit for her to develop.

   A Briefly looking at the feet in good light after bathing or before putting on socks is all that is necessary for foot inspection at this time.

B If SA discovers any foot problems or abnormalities, she should promptly report these to her healthcare provider.

4 Reassure SA that at the present time her risk of foot complications is low. Even if she were to get a foot ulcer, it would probably heal easily.

5 Emphasize that she should continue wearing good shoes with cushioned soles and insoles and have an annual foot exam with testing for neuropathy. Stress the importance of keeping her blood glucose level near normal to also help prevent foot problems from developing.

6 Point out the additional risks of smoking for people with diabetes. Refer SA to a smoking cessation program if she expresses any interest in quitting.

References

1 Ahroni JH, Boyko EJ, Davignon DR, Pecoraro RE. The health and functional status of veterans with diabetes. Diabetes Care. 1994;17:318-321.

2 Bild DE, Selby JV, Sinnock P, Browner WS, Braveman P, Showstack JA. Lower extremity amputation in people with diabetes: epidemiology and prevention. Diabetes Care. 1989;12:24-31.

3 Boulton AJM, Connor H. The diabetic foot 1988. Diabetic Med. 1988;5:796-798.

4 Bowker NH, Pfeifer MA, eds. Levin and O'Neal's The Diabetic Foot. 6th ed. St. Louis: Mosby; 2001:665-675.

5 Ahroni JH, Boyko EJ. Responsiveness of the SF-36 among veterans with diabetes mellitus. J Diabetes Complications. 2000;14:31-39.

6 Most RS, Sinnock P. The epidemiology of lower extremity amputations in diabetic individuals. Diabetes Care. 1983;6:87-91.

7 Nelson RG, Gohdes DM, Everhart JE, et al. Lower extremity amputations in NIDDM: 12-year follow-up study in Pima Indians. Diabetes Care. 1988;11:8-16.

8 Lavery LA, Ashry HR, vanHoutum W, Pugh JA, Harkless LB, Basu S. Variation in the incidence and proportion of diabetes-related amputations in minorities. Diabetes Care. 1996;19:48-52.

9 Selby JV, Zhang D. Risk factors for lower extremity amputation in persons with diabetes. Diabetes Care. 1995;18:509-516.

10 Deerochanawong C, Home PD, Alberti KGMM. A survey of lower limb amputation in diabetic patients. Diabetic Med. 1992;9:942-946.

11 Reiber GE, Boyko EJ, Smith DG. Lower extremity foot ulcers and amputations in diabetes. In: National Diabetes Data Group. Diabetes in America. 2nd ed. Bethesda, Md: National Institutes of Health, National Institute of Diabetes and Digestive and Kidney Disorders; 1995. NIH publication 95-1468:409-428.

12 Pell JP, Donnan PT, Fowkes FG, Ruckley CV. Quality of life following lower limb amputation for peripheral arterial disease. Eur J Vasc Surg. 1993;7:448-451.

13 Reiber GE. Diabetic foot care. Financial implications and practice guidelines. Diabetes Care. 1992;15(suppl 1):29-31.

14 Apelqvist J, Ragnarson-Tennvall G, Larsson J, Persson U. Long-term costs for foot ulcers in diabetic patients in multidisciplinary setting. Foot Ankle Int. 1995;16:388-394.

15 US Department of Health and Human Services. National Hospital Discharge Survey. Hyattsville, Md: National Center for Health Statistics, Centers for Disease Control and Prevention; 1994.

16 Ford ES, Wetterhall SF. The validity of diabetes on hospital discharge diagnoses. Diabetes. 1991;40(suppl 1):449A.

17 Franklin GM, Kahn LB, Baxter J, Marshall JA, Hamman RF. Sensory neuropathy in non-insulin dependent diabetes mellitus. The San Luis Valley Diabetes Study. Am J Epidemiol. 1990;131:633-643.

18 Pecoraro RE, Reiber GE, Burgess EM. Pathways to diabetic limb amputation: basis for prevention. Diabetes Care. 1990;13:513-521.

19 Tanenberg RJ, Schumer MP, Greene DA, Pfeifer MA. Neuropathic problems of the lower extremities in diabetic patients. In: Bowker NH, Pfeifer MA, eds. Levin and O'Neal's The Diabetic Foot. 6th ed. St. Louis: Mosby; 2001:33-64.

20 Holewski JJ, Stess RM, Graf PM, Grunfeld C. Aesthesiometry: quantification of cutaneous pressure sensation in diabetic peripheral neuropathy. J Rehabil Res Dev. 1988; 25:1-10.

21 McNeely MJ, Boyko EJ, Ahroni JH, et al. The independent contribution of diabetic neuropathy and vasculopathy in foot ulceration. How great are the risks? Diabetes Care. 1995;18:216-219.

22 Young MJ, Adams JE, Marshall A, Selby PL, Boulton AJM. Osteopenia, neurological dysfunction and the development of Charcot neuroarthropathy. Diabetes Care. 1995; 18:34-38.

23 Edmonds ME, Roberts VC, Watkins PJ. Blood flow in the diabetic neuropathic foot. Diabetologia. 1982;22:9-15.

24 Flynn MD, Tooke JE. Aetiology of diabetic foot ulceration: a role for the microcirculation. Diabetic Med. 1992;9:320-329.

25 Sanders LJ, Frykberg RG. Diabetic neuropathic osteoarthropathy: the Charcot foot. In: Frykberg RG, ed. The High Risk Foot in Diabetes Mellitus. New York: Churchill-Livingston; 1991:197-338.

26 Lippmann HI, Perotto A, Farrar R. The neuropathic foot of the diabetic. Bull New York Acad Med. 1976;52:1159-1178.

27 Reiber GE. Who is at risk of limb loss and what to do about it. J Rehabil Res Dev. 1994;31:357-362.

28 Palumbo PH, Melton LJ. Peripheral vascular disease and diabetes. In: National Diabetes Data Group. Diabetes in America. 2nd ed. Bethesda, Md: National Institutes of Health, National Institute of Diabetes and Digestive and Kidney Disorders; 1995. NIH publication 95-1468:401-408.

29 Bell DS. Lower limb problems in diabetic patients: what are the causes? What are the remedies? Postgrad Med. 1991;89:237-240,243-244.

30 Pecoraro R. The nonhealing ulcer: a major cause for limb loss. In: Barbul A, Caldwell MD, Eaglestein EH, et al, eds. Clinical and Experimental Approaches to Dermal and Epidermal Repair: Normal and Chronic Wounds. New York: Wiley-Liss; 1991:27-43.

31 Bauman NH, Brand PW. Measurement of pressure between foot and shoe. Lancet. 1963;1:629-632.

32 Pecoraro RE, Ahroni JH, Boyko EJ, Stensel VL. Chronology and determinants of tissue repair in diabetic lower extremity ulcers. Diabetes. 1991;40:1305-1313.

33 Ahroni JH. The care of lower extremity lesions in patients with diabetes. Nurs Pract Forum. 1991;2:188-192.

34 Lipsky BA, Pecoraro RE, Larson SA, Hanley ME, Ahroni JH. Outpatient management of uncomplicated lower-extremity infections in diabetic patients. Arch Intern Med. 1990;150:790-797.

35 Haas LB, Ahroni JH. Lower limb self-management education. In: Bowker NH, Pfeifer MA, eds. Levin and O'Neal's The Diabetic Foot. 6th ed. St. Louis: Mosby; 2001: 665-675.

36 Ahroni JH. Teaching foot care creatively and successfully. Diabetes Educ. 1993;19:320-325.

37 Boyko, EJ, Ahroni JH, Davignon D, Stensel V, Prigeon RL, Smith DG. Diagnostic utililty of the history and physical examination for peripheral vascular disease among patients with diabetes mellitus. J Clin Epidemiol. 1997;50:659-668.

38 Edmonds ME, Blundell MP, Morris ME, Thomas EM, Cotton LT, Watkins PJ. Improved survival of the diabetic foot: the role of a specialized foot clinic. Q J Med. 1986;60:763-771.

Suggested Readings

Ahroni JH. Teaching foot care creatively and successfully. Diabetes Educ. 1993;9:320-325.

Ahroni JH. 101 Foot Care Tips for People With Diabetes. Alexandria, Va: American Diabetes Association; 2000.

Haas LB, Ahroni JH. Lower limb self-management education. In: Bowker NH, Pfeifer MA, eds. Levin and O'Neal's The Diabetic Foot. 6th ed. St. Louis: Mosby; 2001:665-675.

Haas LB. Lower extremity amputations: strategies for prevention. Diabetes Spectrum. 1995;8:206-231.

"Feet Can Last a Lifetime" patient and professional materials available from the National Diabetes Information Clearinghouse (301-654-3327) or on the Internet at: *http://www.niddk.gov* under health information. Accessed November 2000.

"Diabetic Foot Ulcers: A Clinical Practice Guideline" available from the American College of Foot and Ankle Surgeons (800-421-2237) or on the Internet at: *www.diabetes.org/enews/001102_ACF.asp*. Accessed November 2000.

Learning Assessment: Post-Test Questions

Diabetic Foot Care and Education   4

1 Which of the following factors is the most important in maintaining skin integrity of the foot in a person with diabetes?
  A Inspect the feet every day
  B Keep feet germ free with alcohol
  C Wear only white socks with closed-toe shoes
  D Use emollients between the toes to prevent dry, flaky skin

2 To help keep feet warm at night, recommend using:
  A An electric blanket
  B A heating pad
  C A hot water bottle
  D Wool socks

3 A characteristic of foot ulceration is that it:
  A Requires hospitalization
  B Usually involves joint spaces and bone
  C Is usually caused by minor, repetitive pressure
  D May not be preventable in persons with long-standing diabetes

4 The best indicator of peripheral sensory neuropathy is:
  A Intermittent claudication
  B Inability to perceive the 5.07 monofilament
  C Callus over the metatarsal heads
  D Maceration between the toes

5 A sign of peripheral vascular disease is:
  A Cracked, reddened, flaky skin
  B Venous filling time greater than 20 seconds
  C Palpable pedal pulses
  D Prominent metatarsal heads

6 All of the following should be included in every diabetic foot risk screening examination except:
  A Test of foot sensation
  B Palpation of pedal pulses
  C Measure of foot pressure
  D Assessment of foot shape

7 BG was diagnosed with type 2 diabetes 15 years ago. At the time of diagnosis he was told he had "a little sugar and not to worry about it." He has recently retired and seeks your assistance after noting a painless, nonhealing sore on the bottom of his right great toe. BG's right great toe demonstrates significant erythema, edema, increased local warmth, and moderate foul drainage. Based on this description, what BG needs most today is:
  A Diabetes education
  B Segmental Doppler blood pressure studies
  C Antibiotics
  D Protective footwear

8 The director of your facility asks for your opinion on which program is most likely to lower the long-term foot complication and amputation rates in your patient population. Which of the following programs would be most effective?
  A A diabetic foot ulcer clinic for patients with chronic wounds
  B A diabetes foot care education program for people with high-risk feet
  C A comprehensive diabetes care and education program aimed at improving the glycemic control of all people with diabetes
  D A support group for amputees with diabetes

9 The most effective treatment for preventing peripheral vascular disease resulting from arteriosclerosis is:
  A A graduated walking program
  B Angioplasty
  C Cessation of smoking
  D Diuretics to reduce edema

10 Instruct patients with dry, cracked skin on their feet to:
  A Use a callus remover daily
  B Soak feet in warm water daily for 10 to 15 minutes
  C Apply powder or cornstarch after bathing
  D Apply emollients to dry skin of the feet

See next page for answer key.

Post-Test Answer Key

Diabetic Foot Care and Education 4

1	A		**6**	C
2	D		**7**	C
3	C		**8**	C
4	B		**9**	C
5	B		**10**	D

A Core Curriculum for Diabetes Education
Diabetes and Complications

Skin and Dental Care 5

Cheryl Hunt, RN, MSEd, CDE
Health Education and Resources
Alexandria, Virginia

Introduction

1 This chapter on skin and dental care deals with issues of having diabetes and its effect on the skin and its integrity. Understanding the effect of diabetes on the health of the skin, oral mucosa, and teeth is important as educators work with patients with diabetes.

2 Skin, the largest organ of the human body, provides an important defense against infection when it is intact and healthy.

3 Hyperglycemia affects the condition of the skin by contributing to dry skin, rashes, boils, and increased growth of certain bacterial colonies. People with diabetes tend to have a higher risk of lower-extremity and group ß-streptococcal infections than people without diabetes.[1]

4 Hyperglycemia in combination with vascular insufficiency; neuropathy; dry, cracked skin; and/or excoriations caused by pressure or blunt force trauma provides avenues for the sequelae of tissue breakdown, infection, and amputation.[2,3]

5 Controlling blood glucose levels, maintaining adequate nutrition and hydration, and caring for the skin can reduce the risk of infection in people with diabetes.

6 Among people with diabetes, periodontal disease occurs with such frequency and severity that it has been labeled the sixth complication of diabetes mellitus.[4] Although having diabetes and its potential for poor metabolic control is frequently implicated as the cause for periodontal disease, poor oral hygiene is the main cause.

7 Oral hygiene, regular dental care, and improved metabolic control in people with either type 1 or type 2 diabetes reduces the risk of periodontal disease.

Objectives

Upon completion of this chapter, the learner will be able to
1 State the relationship between metabolic control and healthy skin.
2 List 2 elements of effective skin care.
3 Identify the risk associated with loss of metabolic control when infection occurs in people with diabetes.
4 State the relationship between metabolic control and overall dental health.
5 Identify the factors that contribute to periodontal disease in people with diabetes.
6 List 2 effective dental care practices.

Diabetes and Skin Disease

1 Dry skin may occur more frequently in people with diabetes.
   A Hyperglycemia resulting in polyuria may be a cause of dehydration and subsequent dry skin.
   B *Anhidrosis,* which is defined as an autonomic neuropathic condition of diabetes in which little or no perspiration is produced in the feet and legs, may lead to drying and cracking of the skin.

C Elevated blood glucose levels and impaired circulation increase the risk of infection and present a situation of serious concern if either of the previous two circumstances are present.

2 People with poorly controlled diabetes complicated by vascular or neuropathic changes demonstrate an increased risk for skin infection caused by staphylococci, ß-hemolytic streptococci, and fungus.

3 Common infections of the skin that have a probable relationship to diabetes are
  A Cutaneous infections: furunculosis and carbuncles
  B Candida: affecting areas of the genitalia, upper thighs, and under the breast
  C Cellulitis and/or lower-extremity vascular ulcers[5]

4 Infections usually increase the blood glucose level and, consequently, the patient's insulin requirements.

5 Maintaining metabolic control is important for both preventing and treating skin problems.

6 Cleanliness, adequate nutrition with appropriate consumption of fluids, and avoiding trauma to the skin are important components of care that help to maintain skin integrity and prevent infection. In addition using a mild soap, warm (not hot) water, moisturizing lotion (not oil-based and without alcohol), and sunscreen help to maintain healthy skin.

Diabetes and Dental Care

1 *Periodontal disease*, an inflammatory process that affects the supporting tissues of the teeth, may be accelerated in people with diabetes that is poorly controlled or of long duration.[6-8]
  A Periodontal disease is the most prevalent oral complication of diabetes.
  B Factors responsible for or contributing to the development of periodontal disease are
    • Basement membrane thickening
    • Possible changes in vasculature
    • Changes in the microflora of periodontal tissues
    • Impaired collagen metabolism
    • Impaired leukocyte function and other aspects of the host response[6,9]
  C Because periodontal disease is often asymptomatic, people may have a false sense of dental health.[9]

2 Caries in the crown of a tooth seems to occur with greater frequency in adults with poorly controlled diabetes.[6] Hyperglycemia may contribute to elevated salivary glucose levels, which increase the risk of developing periodontal disease and dental caries.

3 Oral infections other than dental caries or periodontal disease are often more severe in people with poorly controlled diabetes than those with well-controlled diabetes or those who do not have diabetes.[6]

4 Insulin doses may need to be adjusted depending upon the degree of periodontal health.

A Infection may increase insulin requirements.

B Controlling infection and maintaining oral health may reduce insulin requirements.

5 Dental care and metabolic control contribute to the prevention of dental caries and periodontal disease.[6,9]

A Bacterial plaque must be kept at a minimum.

• Instruct patients to routinely brush and floss teeth.

• Professional removal of plaque should be done periodically in association with regular dental exams.

• The use of baking soda with hydrogen peroxide has been identified as being helpful in the eradication of subgingival microflora.

B During routine medical visits, people with diabetes need to be assessed for signs of redness, foul odor, swelling, bleeding, loose teeth, or pain; offer appropriate referral if these periodontal symptoms develop. Instruct patients to see a dentist every 6 months, and more frequently if periodontal disease exists.

Key Educational Considerations

1 Inform people with diabetes who have obvious signs of dry skin or compromised skin integrity about the risk of infection and further deterioration of the skin. Part of the information should be a reminder that armpits, the space between fingers and toes, around the nails, and other moist areas promote growth of fungi.

2 Emphasize the importance of metabolic control, cleanliness, moisturization, skin assessment, and reporting of problem areas to the diabetes care team.

3 Advise patients to avoid trauma to the skin, especially the feet and legs. Use of properly fitting shoes and socks, protective sporting equipment when exercising, and general caution during routine daily activities can help reduce the risk of trauma to the skin. Poor metabolic control also causes dry, itchy skin, which may lead to scratching and irritation, issuing an invitation to an invasion of bacteria.

4 Teach people with diabetes to

A Bathe or cleanse skin with warm water and mild soap.

B Avoid overexposure to water or cleansing products because these may strip the skin of its normal protective oils.

C Pat skin dry with a soft, fluffy towel rather than rubbing it with the towel.

D Thoroughly dry the skin between skin folds and toes. Powders or cornstarch may be applied to keep moist areas dry. Dry skin may be moistened with lanolin or hand lotion, but should not be used excessively. Lotions containing alcohol are not suitable as the alcohol may contribute to drying or cracking of the skin.

E Follow a balanced nutritional plan with appropriate liquid consumption.

5 Approach issues of skin and dental care in a nonjudgmental way, maintaining sensitivity to individual and cultural differences.

A Present accurate information that will reinforce the importance of self-care to lower risks while reducing unrealistic fears.

B Apprehension associated with dental examinations and treatment can be reduced by explaining what to expect and by reinforcing the positive outcomes of dental care.

6 Stress the importance of preventing dental complications through routine dental examinations, effective brushing and flossing, and keeping blood glucose levels near normal.

7 Advise persons taking insulin secretagogues or insulin to schedule dental appointments about 1 hour after a meal to reduce the chances of hypoglycemia. When anesthesia is to be used, inform patients that the best outcome may be facilitated by having the dentist or oral surgeon collaborate with their doctor or nurse practitioner.

8 Nutritional modification and appropriate instruction may be necessary for preventing and/or treating periodontal disease. Instruction may focus on eating a balanced food plan, decreasing intake of sugars, ingesting important vitamins and minerals, and making changes to accommodate treatments or impaired ability to chew foods.

9 Be prepared to recommend dentists or local dental clinics for people who have not established a program of routine dental care.

Self-Review Questions

1 Describe the best preventive measures for dental problems in people with diabetes.

2 State why products for the skin containing alcohol should be avoided.

Learning Assessment: Case Study 1

TL is a 63-year-old female with an 8-year history of type 2 diabetes. She has tried a variety of oral medications to control her blood glucose, with little success. TL's blood glucose levels remain elevated in the range of 220 mg/dL to 280 mg/dL for no obvious reason. Today you notice that her gums are unusually red and you detect a foul breath odor as she speaks to you. Further questioning reveals that TL has recently had to alter her eating habits to soft foods because her mouth has been so tender and her gums bleed so easily. TL tells you she fears the dentist and she has not seen one in the past 4 years.

Questions for Discussion

1 How could infection in the gingiva affect TL's blood glucose levels?

2 What are age-appropriate concerns related to TL's oral health?

3 What aspects of personal oral hygiene are important to discuss with TL?

4 Who are possible professional referrals you can offer to TL?

Discussion

1 Periodontal disease may be responsible for TL's persistently elevated blood glucose levels that have failed to respond to pharmacologic therapy. In addition, elevated blood glucose levels increase the risk for periodontal disease.

2 Teach TL about the various aspects of oral hygiene and how dental problems such as periodontal disease can affect blood glucose levels.

3 She should be given referrals to appropriate dental health professionals (a dentist, periodontist, or oral surgeon) to treat her oral health problems while she continues to work with her diabetes care team to lower her blood glucose levels.

4 Given the relationship between her age, current state of dental health, and glycemic control, the following outcomes should be considered:
   A Impact of loss of teeth, soreness, and/or infection in the oral cavity
   B Influence of normal changes in taste and smell on her willingness to use a meal plan as part of her diabetes care

References

1 Boyko EJ, Lipsky BA. Infection and diabetes. In: National Diabetes Data Group, eds. Diabetes in America. 2nd ed. Bethesda, Md: National Institutes of Health; 1995. NIH publication 95-1468:485-500.

2 Reeves WG, Wilson RM. Infection, immunity, and diabetes. In: Alberti KGMM, DeFronzo RA, Keen H, Zimmet P, eds. International Textbook of Diabetes Mellitus. New York: John Wiley & Sons; 1992:1165-1171.

3 Pecoraro RE, Reiber GE, Burgess EM. Pathways to diabetic limb amputation. Basis for prevention. Diabetes Care. 1990;13:513-521.

4 Loe H. Periodontal disease. The sixth complication of diabetes mellitus. Diabetes Care. 1993;16:329-334.

5 American Diabetes Association. Detection and treatment of complications. In: Medical Management of Type 2 Diabetes. 4th ed. Alexandria, Va: American Diabetes Association; 1998:100-134.

6 Loe H, Genco RJ. Oral complications in diabetes. In: National Diabetes Data Group, eds. Diabetes in America. 2nd ed. Bethesda, Md: National Institutes of Health; 1995. NIH publication 95-1468:501-506.

7 Sznajder N, Carraro JJ, Rugna S, Sereday M. Periodontal findings in diabetic and non-diabetic patients. J Clin Periodont. 1978;49:445-448.

8 Hugoson A, Thorstennson H, Falk H, Kuylenstierna J. Periodontal conditions in insulin-dependent diabetics. J Clin Periodont. 1989;16:215-223.

9 Hallmon W, Measley BL. Implications of diabetes mellitus and periodontal disease. Diabetes Educ. 1992;18:310-315.

Suggested Readings

Betschart JM, Betschart JE. Periodontal disease and diabetes mellitus. Diabetes Spectrum. 1997;2:112-118.

Holdren RD, Patton LL. Oral conditions associated with diabetes mellitus. Diabetes Spectrum. 1993;6:11-17.

Stillman N, Genco RJ. Periodontal disease and diabetes interdependent conditions. Practical Diabetology. 2000;Dec:19-27.

Learning Assessment: Post-Test Questions

Skin and Dental Care

5

1 Which of the following factors is the most important in maintaining skin integrity in a person with diabetes?
   A Avoid exposure to sun
   B Maintain blood glucose levels within target ranges
   C Wear only white socks with closed toed shoes
   D Use oil-based creams to prevent dry, flaky skin

2 In addition to elevated blood glucose levels, a reason that people with diabetes may be at increased risk for infection is
   A Impaired circulation
   B Excessive perspiration
   C Anhidrosis
   D Overuse of oil-based lotions

3 Common pathogens causing skin infections in people with diabetes include all except
   A ß–hemolytic streptococci
   B Fungus
   C Haemophilus influenzae type b
   D Staphylococci

4 All of the following negatively impact dental health except
   A Hyperglycemia
   B Excessive production of saliva
   C Basement membrane thickening
   D Dental plaque

See next page for answer key.

Post-Test Answer Key

Skin and Dental Care   5

1   B

2   A

3   C

4   B

A Core Curriculum for Diabetes Education
Diabetes and Complications

Macrovascular Disease 6

Frank Vinicor, MD, MPH
Centers for Disease Control and Prevention
Division of Diabetes Translation
Atlanta, Georgia

Introduction

1 In the United States and throughout the world, the prevalence of diabetes is increasing at epidemic rates[1-3] and the onset of diabetes, including type 2, is occurring at younger ages.[4] Unless the gap between what is known to be effective therapy and what is actually done in daily medical practices is narrowed,[5] the number of diabetes-associated complications can be expected to increase substantially.[6]

2 Among the many conditions associated with diabetes, cardiovascular diseases (CVD) are the most frequent, serious, lethal, and costly.[7-10] In the 1990s, important scientific understanding emerged about diabetes-related CVD and clear evidence that the CVD burden of diabetes can be reduced and controlled using the knowledge we have today.

A *Arteriosclerosis* is a general term that describes the condition in which the walls of blood vessels (both arteries and veins) are thick, hard, and nonelastic.

B *Atherosclerosis* is a specific term that refers to the process of materials being deposited along and within blood vessel walls (especially arterial).

C *Macrovascular disease* is a term that refers to both arteriosclerotic and atherosclerotic changes in moderate-sized to large-sized arteries and veins. Coronary, cerebral, and peripheral macrovascular diseases are particularly significant because of the associated frequency, morbidity, and mortality and because of their economic consequences.[7-11]

3 Atherosclerosis, which is common in diabetes, is literally a "soft" hardening in which mounds of lipid material mixed with smooth muscle cells and calcium accumulate in the inner walls of blood vessels. These mounds, called *plaques,* become enlarged over time.

A Eventually the plaque may block blood flow, weaken, and rupture its contents into the blood stream and/or cause the formation of a blood clot.

B Plaques may also initiate vascular spasm, which further reduces blood flow.

C Plaque formations occur by several different mechanisms.[12,13]

- Smooth muscle cells, which normally lie behind the inner wall, or intima, of a blood vessel may migrate into this intima, spread across its surface, and form the base of plaque. What starts this process of migration is not known for certain. Injury to the intima may initiate this smooth muscle migration, with the injury itself reflecting mechanical insult, oxygen deficiency, or lipid deposition. As the plaque forms, cholesterol becomes a major component.

- Calcium deposits may also cause further hardening of plaque.

- All plaques are not the same, and recent investigations[13] identified vulnerable, thinly capped plaques, which are common in diabetes mellitus, as being associated with greater morbidity and mortality than stable plaques with a thick fibrous cap over the fatty compartment.

- The concept of *vulnerable plaque* is substantially changing views of the pathogenesis of cardiac ischemia from one of a defect in anatomy (eg, blockage in flow) to a biological event (eg, rupture and clot formation resulting in flow impairment).[14,15]

Objectives

Upon completion of this chapter, the learner will be able to

1 Identify the types of macrovascular disease that occur among persons with diabetes mellitus.

2 Explain the contribution of macrovascular disease to the overall disease and economic burden associated with diabetes mellitus.

3 Describe special features of macrovascular disease in persons with diabetes, including pathogenesis, clinical manifestations, detection, and treatment.

4 Identify risk factors that may contribute to the prevalence, morbidity, and mortality of macrovascular disease in diabetes.

5 Describe assessment and intervention strategies that prevent and/or minimize macrovascular disease in diabetes mellitus.

Types of Macrovascular Disease That Affect Persons With Diabetes

1 The 3 major types of macrovascular disease are coronary artery, cerebral vascular, and peripheral vascular disease.[8-10]

  A In persons with diabetes, most studies indicate that atherosclerotic vascular disease of the coronary vessels develops at an earlier age than in the nondiabetic population and involves coronary vessels more extensively and diffusely.

  - The incidence of early-onset or midlife atherosclerotic coronary artery disease (CAD) is relatively comparable in men and women with diabetes but much lower among nondiabetic women than nondiabetic men. What this means is that women with diabetes lose their gender protection from atherosclerosis.[16,17]

  - The adverse consequences of an acute coronary event (eg, sudden death, heart failure, arrhythmia) and the likelihood of a recurrent myocardial infarction are greater in persons with diabetes.[18-22]

  B Persons with diabetes appear to be prone to cerebral vascular disease developing at an earlier age than nondiabetic individuals. (The data are not quite as strong or extensive for diabetes-related cerebral vascular disease when compared with diabetes-associated coronary artery disease.) Persons with diabetes also seem to be at risk for both transient ischemic attacks and thrombotic cerebral vascular accidents.[23]

  C Peripheral vascular disease (PVD) is very common in persons with diabetes, especially those with long-standing disease, and is clinically characterized by intermittent claudication, lower-leg and vascular foot ulcers, and often the need for amputations. Smoking, dyslipidemia, hypertension, and other conditions such as peripheral neuropathy may contribute to the progression or clinical expression of peripheral vascular disease.

2 Complications associated with macrovascular disease contribute significantly to the morbidity, disability, mortality, and costs associated with diabetes, particularly in those persons with long-standing diabetes.[8-10]

  A Most clinical and epidemiological studies[6,7] show that coronary artery disease accounts for 50% to 60% of all deaths in patients with diabetes. In recent studies, individuals with diabetes without a clinically apparent myocardial infarction had a mortality rate similar to nondiabetic individuals who already had experienced and survived a heart attack.[24]

- Persons with type 2 diabetes are particularly at risk for coronary-associated mortality as well as for various morbid consequences of coronary ischemia.[6,7] Coronary artery disease is also the greatest cause of mortality in persons with type 1 diabetes.[25] Over the past 2 to 3 decades there has been a continued reduction in mortality from CVD among persons without diabetes. In contrast, however, mortality rates from CVD among men with diabetes have not decreased, and the rates in women with diabetes may be increasing.[26]
- In general, mortality ratios for coronary artery disease in persons with diabetes are twofold and fourfold greater in men and women with diabetes, respectively, than in a comparable nondiabetic population.[27]

B Most persons with diabetes who experience acute coronary insufficiency display usual symptoms of acute coronary ischemia (eg, angina, diaphoresis, anxiety, shortness of breath). However, an important element of coronary artery disease in patients with diabetes is the so-called silent or atypical myocardial infarction, in which patients do not manifest the typical symptoms of acute coronary ischemia.

- Although the data are controversial, most studies suggest that silent myocardial infarctions are more common in persons with diabetes than in those without diabetes, especially if the diabetes is of long-standing duration.
- Because of autonomic neuropathy, symptoms such as nausea, shortness of breath, sweating, and vomiting may be present rather than angina.
- Sudden death outside the hospital setting may occur at greater rates among those with diabetes than in the nondiabetic population.[28]
- When assessing patients' symptoms in activities such as exercise programs, silent coronary artery disease and possible atypical manifestations of coronary artery disease should be considered.

C There is little relationship between the duration of type 2 diabetes and the presence of coronary events. Individuals with impaired glucose tolerance have CVD morbidity and mortality rates similar to those with established diabetes[29] (see discussion in this chapter concerning impaired glucose tolerance, the metabolic syndrome, and improper intrauterine nutrition for possible explanations). For persons with type 1 diabetes, however, the longer the duration of diabetes, the more likely it is that the person will experience a coronary event.

D Studies of cerebral vascular disease in persons with diabetes are limited but suggest that mortality ratios are from 3 to 5 times greater than for the nondiabetic population.

- There is a relationship between the level of glycemic control at admission for a stroke in persons with diabetes and subsequent mortality.[30]
- The increased likelihood of cerebral vascular death applies to both men and women.

E Peripheral vascular disease infrequently leads to fatal complications during the first few years after clinical expression. Thus, most epidemiologic investigations are based on nonfatal complications, symptoms, or clinical findings associated with peripheral vascular disease (see Chapter 4, Diabetic Foot Care and Education, in Diabetes and Complications, for more information about lower-extremity complications). Approximately 50% of all nontraumatic lower-extremity amputations in the United States are performed on persons with diabetes and are due primarily to peripheral neuropathy but also peripheral vascular disease. People with diabetes have a 15 times higher age-related risk for amputation than nondiabetic individuals.[31]

- Absent peripheral pulses due to occlusive peripheral arterial disease are seen considerably more often in patients with type 2 diabetes than in patients with type 1 diabetes.
- The incidence of occlusive peripheral arterial disease is approximately 4 to 6 times higher in men and women with diabetes, respectively, than in those without diabetes.[31] Thus, the need for preventive education about foot care is particularly important in persons with diabetes. Recent health services research studies of the diabetic foot support this need for foot care education.[31]

Magnitude of the Problem

1 Determining how common, serious, and costly a diabetes complication is assists in characterizing and describing the dimension of the disease problem. Further, understanding the magnitude and nature of a problem facilitates a better understanding of how likely various interventions can reduce the diabetes burden.

   A Of the approximately 190 000 deaths in 1995 for which diabetes was listed as an underlying or contributing factor, almost 125 000 were due to CAD.[32]

   B The greatest cause of mortality among persons with either type 1 or type 2 diabetes is cardiovascular disease (CVD), with 61% of premature deaths due to a combination of CVD and cerebral vascular disease.[33] These data likely underestimate the true contribution of CVD to diabetes mortality because of the continued inaccuracy of death certificates among persons with known diabetes.[34]

2 Regarding health resource utilization (eg, hospitalizations, clinic visits), PVD and CVD accounted for approximately 26% of all days in the hospital and hospital discharges among those with diabetes in 1997.[7,11] Furthermore, 15% of the almost 70 million nursing home days for persons with diabetes were due to the sequelae of cerebral and cardiovascular disease, and 6% of the over 30 million physician visits for persons with diabetes in 1997 were primarily for assessment of cerebral vascular and cardiovascular disease.[7,11]

3 In terms of costs, almost 20% of the $44 billion healthcare expenditures in 1997 directly attributable to diabetes were for cardiovascular and peripheral vascular disease.[11] Furthermore, 58% of mortality costs attributable to diabetes in 1997 reflect premature death in persons with diabetes due to either cerebral vascular or cardiovascular disease.[11]

4 CVD is thus the most lethal, devastating, and costly complication of diabetes and a major factor in loss of quality of life among persons with diabetes. Even small risk reductions in diabetes-associated cardiovascular disease would have a substantial impact on the overall diabetes burden. Given interventional science concerning diabetes-associated CVD that has accumulated over the past 5 years, there is reason for optimism that the overall burden of diabetes can be substantially controlled by improving the translation of science into daily clinical and public health practices.

Risk Factors for Cardiovascular Disease

1 A large number of risk factors may contribute to the accelerated atherosclerotic vascular disease in patients with diabetes, including lipid abnormalities, hypertension, smoking, obesity, physical inactivity, nutrition, hyperinsulinemia, insulin resistance, blood flow dynamics and coagulation factors, albuminuria, hyperglycemia per se, and some past treatment approaches and medications.[35] By using data about the presence of these risk factors, it is possible to establish risk stratification tables for CVD among persons with diabetes.[36]

A Abnormal lipid levels and types of lipids, such as elevated plasma triglyceride and lowered high-density lipoprotein (HDL) levels, are often found in patients with insulin resistance, impaired glucose tolerance, and type 2 diabetes. Total cholesterol and low-density lipoprotein (LDL) cholesterol levels are generally comparable between persons with type 2 diabetes and matched nondiabetic individuals. In persons with well-controlled type 1 diabetes, lipoprotein levels are similar to control subjects. Qualitative abnormalities in lipid components have also been identified in persons with diabetes, including very dense lipoproteins and increased amounts of lipoprotein Lp(a).[37,38] These qualitative abnormalities in lipid subfractions may contribute significantly to accelerated CVD among persons with diabetes.

- There remains some controversy regarding whether elevated triglycerides are an independent risk factor for coronary artery disease, both in the general population and in persons with diabetes.[39] However, evidence is accumulating that controlling triglycerides is important for those with diabetes.[40] Postprandial elevations of triglycerides in the form of chylomicrons, and perhaps postmeal hyperglycemia, may be particularly serious.[41,42]

- Plasma triglyceride levels correlate positively with blood glucose and glycosylated hemoglobin levels. In both type 1 and type 2 patients, improved metabolic control results in lowered triglyceride levels and some minimal degree of reciprocal increase in HDL levels.

- The impact of plasma cholesterol levels on the subsequent development of cardiovascular disease is probably similar in individuals with and without diabetes. Thus, if an elevated cholesterol level doubles the chance of a myocardial infarction in a nondiabetic individual, a similar cholesterol level will likely have a comparable effect in a person with diabetes.[36]

- Persons with diabetes seem to start from a higher baseline regarding mortality from CVD in the absence of other risk factors (eg, cholesterol, hypertension), perhaps as a direct result of the effect of diabetes on vascular endothelial function.[43] The deleterious interaction of the several risk factors for macrovascular disease may also be present for several years before the onset of hyperglycemia, thus contributing to the appearance of accelerated CVD among persons with diabetes.[44] In addition, the qualitative nature of lipid structures (eg, greater density of lipid particles, glycosylation, and/or oxidation of lipoproteins) may be as important as the absolute levels.

- In both type 1 and type 2 diabetes, the correlation between hyperglycemia and HDL levels is poor, suggesting a complex interrelationship (ie, achieving glycemic control, by itself, will not necessarily substantially increase HDL levels).

- Effective and safe ways to increase HDL levels need to be identified because low HDL levels are a powerful and independent predictor of subsequent vascular events.[37,38]

B Elevated plasma fibrinogen levels and other indicators of defective clotting dynamics exist in diabetes and appear to be strongly associated with diabetic macrovascular disease.[9,15] In recent epidemiologic studies in the general population, an elevated plasma fibrinogen level was identified as a potent risk factor for future cardiovascular morbidity and mortality. Both cigarette smoking and hyperglycemia raise fibrinogen levels, thus underscoring the importance of smoking cessation and glycemic control in the possible prevention of coronary disease. Elevated fibrinogen levels may be a component of an activated inflammatory process that is present among persons with and without diabetes with pending and existing CVD.[45,46] For example, C-reactive protein and other inflammatory markers have been shown to be associated with an increased incidence of acute coronary events. Whether these markers of inflammation are primary or secondary, they underscore the importance of aspirin therapy in persons with diabetes.

C Hypertension is approximately twice as common in persons with diabetes than in nondiabetic individuals. Hypertension is an independent risk factor for cardiovascular disease in the general population as well as in patients with diabetes. Recent therapeutic interventions for hypertension among persons with diabetes and hypertension documented an impressive reduction in CVD mortality and morbidity with even modest improvements in hypertension.[47] The improvement in CVD mortality and morbidity among persons with diabetes seems to be related to how low the blood pressure can be safely reduced.[48] Use of an angiotensin-converting enzyme inhibitor among persons with diabetes and no clinical CVD has been shown to reduce subsequent CVD events.[49] These interventional studies highlight the importance of focusing more attention on hypertension treatment among persons with diabetes.

- In type 1 diabetes there is a correlation between duration of diabetes, the presence of renal dysfunction, and the development of hypertension. In both type 1 and type 2 diabetes there is a strong association between a common marker of renal disease, microalbuminuria and macroalbuminuria, and subsequent mortality from CVD.[50]

- In persons with type 2 diabetes, the pathogenesis of hypertension may be associated with the *metabolic syndrome* (also called insulin resistance syndrome or syndrome X). In this syndrome, at least 4 elements are commonly seen together in clinical practice: hyperglycemia, hyperlipidemia, hypertension, and central obesity.[51] A central role of insulin resistance and subsequent hyperinsulinemia and hypertension, even prior to the onset of hyperglycemia, has been proposed. An atherosclerotic environment may exist for years before the onset of hyperglycemia, including during a time of impaired glucose tolerance.[29] This scenario would explain the lack of a time relationship between the onset of hyperglycemia, hypertension, and CVD in persons with type 2 diabetes. Even among persons with nondiabetic blood glucose and glycosylated hemoglobin levels, there is a direct relationship between the glycemic values and subsequent CVD events.[52] These observational studies indicate that in the future, the diagnostic fasting plasma glucose level may need to be lower than 126 mg/dL (7.0 mmol/L) if CVD disease in persons with diabetes is to be identified and controlled.[53]

- Recent studies indicate that an impaired intrauterine nutritional environment associated with a smaller fetus and newborn also is associated with a high likelihood of developing the metabolic syndrome, coronary artery disease, and type 2 diabetes many decades later.[54,55] This concept may both explain the common association between elements of the metabolic syndrome and offer opportunities for interventions that subsequently prevent and control type 2 diabetes in later life by insuring proper nutrition during pregnancy.

D Persons with diabetes smoke tobacco, on average, at the same frequency as the general population. Unfortunately, younger people with diabetes smoke more often than their nondiabetic peers.[56] Smoking appears to have an independent additive impact on the risk of subsequent cardiovascular disease developing in persons with diabetes and appears also to be associated with an increased incidence of type 2 diabetes[57] and impaired glucose tolerance.[58]

- It is unclear whether the mechanisms for the effects of smoking on vascular function in persons with diabetes are due to cigarette toxins or are mediated through lowered HDL levels or elevated fibrinogen levels.
- Smoking, like diabetes, is associated with an increase in protein glycosylation, including advanced glycosylated end products (AGEs).[59] Thus, the combination of having diabetes and smoking cigarettes could result in a substantial increase in permanent protein glycosylation and subsequent microvascular dysfunction.

E Obesity is a problem for most persons with either impaired glucose tolerance or type 2 diabetes. The independent contribution of obesity to atherosclerotic vascular disease in these patients has not yet been established, perhaps because these same individuals also often have dyslipidemia and/or hypertension.

F Little direct information is presently available on the relationship between physical activity and the risk of atherosclerotic vascular disease among persons with diabetes. Recent studies confirmed a strong association between physical activity and subsequent CVD events, at least among women with diabetes.[60] Whether such a relationship exists in men with diabetes, and/or will be confirmed in a randomized interventional trial, remains to be established. Nevertheless, a well-planned cardiovascular exercise program, with thorough cardiovascular assessment prior to exercise, is a prudent adjunct to therapy for hyperglycemia.[61] Lifestyle and behavioral interventions, including physical activity, are presently being studied to determine whether a reduction in the progression of impaired glucose tolerance to type 2 diabetes will occur.[62]

G Components of the diet may be associated with subsequent CVD. For example, the glycemic index,[63] alcohol consumption,[64] and a diet high in saturated fat and cholesterol may be associated with CVD, but it has been difficult to establish these factors as independent causative agents (see Chapter 1, Medical Nutrition Therapy, in Diabetes Management Therapies, for more information).

H Because blood coagulation factors are important in the formation and dissolution of arterial thrombi, they may contribute to both acute and chronic atherosclerotic lesions. A number of platelet and clotting-factor abnormalities have been reported in persons with diabetes. Platelet behavior tends to improve with better metabolic control.[65] The impact of these coagulation factors underscores the concern about the underuse of aspirin therapy among persons with diabetes who are at risk for CVD.[66]

I Both microalbuminuria and macroalbuminuria appear to be highly associated with the incidence and mortality of macrovascular disease. Whether albuminuria is a risk marker for macrovascular disease (ie, not causative) or a true risk factor is not clear.[50]

J In the past, attention has been directed to a possible role of particular therapeutic agents used to treat diabetes and associated conditions in the pathogenesis of macrovascular disease.

- While results from the University Group Diabetes Program (UGDP) suggested an increased risk of cardiovascular complications in patients with diabetes who were treated with an oral antidiabetes drug, subsequent overall experience with sulfonylureas as well as newer oral agents does not support this association.[67]

- In nondiabetic subjects, hyperinsulinemia is associated with increased risk of coronary artery disease.[68] Some clinical studies of patients with type 2 diabetes suggest that high plasma insulin levels may also be associated with atherosclerotic vascular disease.[69] However, there is considerable controversy regarding the relationships among insulin resistance, hyperinsulinemia, and macrovascular disease in diabetes, including the validity of the insulin assays. At present, no firm and convincing evidence exists that exogenous insulin causes atherosclerosis.

- In the treatment of hypertension, concern has been expressed that side effects from certain antihypertensive agents (eg, diuretics, ß-blockers, calcium-channel blockers) may attenuate, if not reverse, the benefits of blood-pressure-lowering medications theoretically, in part, by increasing insulin resistance or adversely affecting lipid metabolism. Although blood pressure medication must be selected carefully for persons with diabetes, it is very important to establish normal blood pressure in this population.[70,71] It may be more important to be sure that all patients with diabetes and hypertension receive antihypertensive medications than which medication they receive.[72] Thus, given cost considerations and effectiveness, ß-blockers and low-dose thiazide diuretics can be considered as initial therapy.

K Because hyperglycemia is the hallmark of diabetes, the possible contribution of chronically elevated levels of blood glucose to the development of atherosclerotic vascular disease must be considered.

- With hyperglycemia, sorbitol accumulates in the intima of the vascular system and causes this layer to enlarge, possibly contributing to atherosclerotic plaque formation.

- In an environment of hyperglycemia, protein glycosylation within the artery wall may contribute to atherosclerotic vascular disease by altering the normal protein function within the intima.

- Red blood cell deformability and oxygen release are reduced when diabetes is poorly controlled, interfering with tissue oxygen delivery and affecting blood flow.

- Problems with the oxidative state in association with hyperglycemia may also contribute to tissue damage, perhaps through abnormal mitochondrial function.[73]

- At present, several observational studies have demonstrated an association between glycemia and atherosclerosis.[74,75] However, in more rigorous scientific studies such as the Diabetes Control and Complications Trial,[76] the Kumanoto study,[77] and the recently completed UKPDS,[67] the benefits of glucose reduction on macrovascular events were not confirmed. Preliminary and nonstatistical results from the pilot Veterans Administration study[78] suggest, but clearly do not establish, a potential deleterious effect of improved glucose control on atherosclerotic events. The atherogenic process may have begun well before the hyperglycemia began (eg, during insulin resistance or impaired glucose tolerance)[29,51,68] so that glucose control is a very late intervention for atherosclerosis.

2 A number of risk factors may account for excessive macrovascular disease in diabetes. However, their exact individual or aggregate roles are unclear. It is likely that each risk factor for macrovascular disease contributes to the overall prevalence of coronary artery, cerebral vascular, and peripheral vascular disease, and each offers an opportunity to intervene to reduce the burden of CVD among persons with diabetes. Thus, it is important to ensure that risk factor reduction for CVD remains a primary goal of diabetes management for all persons with diabetes who thereby are at risk for CVD.

A The strength of the relationship between the 3 major risk factors—elevated plasma cholesterol level, high blood pressure, and smoking—and the development of atherosclerotic vascular disease is probably the same in persons with diabetes and comparable individuals without diabetes.

B Studies indicate, however, that only a modest proportion of the excess atherosclerotic vascular disease seen in diabetes can be explained by the levels of the general risk factors for vascular disease. Excess atherosclerotic vascular disease in persons with diabetes is probably due to the effects of hyperglycemia through a substantial number of mechanisms and/or other unidentified factors.

- Homocysteine is an amino acid that may affect vascular disease[41] and may be involved in CVD among persons with diabetes.[79,80]

C Achieving and maintaining better glycemic control can improve some of these problems. Recent interventional trials in hypertension and lipid reduction indicate that blood pressure and lipid control are very important among persons with diabetes.

Assessment of Atherosclerotic Vascular Disease

1 The goals of assessment are to (1) determine if clinical manifestations of CVD are present and (2) identify risk factors beyond diabetes that increase the likelihood of developing CVD. Knowing the current nature and extent of disease can be useful for developing secondary prevention programs.

2 The medical history should focus on coronary symptoms (eg, angina, dyspnea), cerebral symptoms (eg, dizziness, transient weakness), and/or peripheral vascular symptoms (eg, claudication, foot ulcers). If symptoms are present, a more extensive history of precipitating and alleviating circumstances should be obtained. The presence of risk factors such as smoking, family history of atherosclerotic vascular disease, personal history of elevated cholesterol levels or blood pressure readings, etc, should also be noted.

3 The physical assessment includes blood pressure measurement (at least 2 measurements either lying or sitting); evaluation for the presence of vascular bruits in the neck, abdomen, and groin; and determination of the status of the feet, including peripheral pulses and evaluation of orthostatic hypotension.

4 Laboratory assessment includes measures of glycemic control, a lipid profile (total cholesterol, HDL cholesterol, LDL cholesterol, triglycerides), and determination of renal function including urinary protein. A baseline EKG and in some circumstances, a stress EKG, can be considered.[81] While electron-beam computed tomography to detect coronary vessel calcification may be useful in the near future for evaluating atherosclerosis, additional study is required.[82]

5 The educational and psychosocial assessments focus on food/nutrition and exercise/physical activity habits; coping skills; smoking; and relevant knowledge, beliefs, attitudes.

Intervention Strategies

1 Because macrovascular disease accounts for such significant morbidity, mortality, and costs among persons with diabetes, therapeutic measures to reduce atherosclerotic risk are imperative. In general, efforts to accomplish this risk reduction can be classified in the following 3 ways:

A Primary: preventive strategies used to decrease the incidence or onset of cardio-vascular disease, symptomatic or asymptomatic

B Secondary: preventive strategies employed after the onset of clinical cardiovascular disease

C Tertiary: intervention strategies used in association with an acute event (eg, myocardial infarction)

2 Primary and secondary interventions for persons with diabetes are very similar and include aggressive treatment of hypertension, cessation of cigarette smoking, reduction in possible coagulation tendencies, treatment of hyperlipidemia, and optimal control of hyperglycemia.

A All of these strategies are designed to slow the development and/or progression of atherosclerotic disease. Of particular importance is the possibility that extensive CVD exists in persons with diabetes even prior to the onset of a clinical event. Thus, data indicate that mortality in persons with diabetes but without clinical CVD is comparable to death rates in persons without diabetes who have already experienced at least 1 coronary event.[24] These initial observations suggest that all persons with diabetes may benefit from preventive strategies for CVD, even in the absence of clinical manifestations of CVD.[83]

B Several recent studies that included persons with diabetes provided convincing evidence of the benefits of lipid and blood pressure control in significantly reducing subsequent CVD events, including mortality.[84-87]

C Underlying each of these medical prevention strategies is critical self-management education, medical nutrition therapy, and physical activity.[42] Meal planning for reduction of saturated fat and cholesterol intake and modest weight loss are some of the important strategies that can be presented to patients as therapeutic options (see Chapter 1, Medical Nutrition Therapy for Diabetes, and Chapter 2, Exercise, in Diabetes Management Therapies, and Chapter 2, Hyperglycemia, in Diabetes and Complications, for more information about these topics).

3 There are several generally accepted principles regarding the treatment of hypertension in persons with diabetes.

A Pharmacologic treatment is likely to be initiated in persons with diabetes who have only modest elevations of blood pressure compared with the general population. In a few studies, persons with diabetes benefited more from a progressive reduction in blood pressure.[88]

B The selection of initial antihypertensive agents for persons with diabetes may differ from the selection for nondiabetic individuals because of the presence of diabetes.
  • Angiotensin-converting enzyme (ACE) inhibitors or calcium-channel blockers are often selected as initial therapy, in part because of apparent beneficial effects on kidney function.

- Low-dose thiazide and/or ß-blockers are also reasonable as first-line therapy. While thiazide diuretics potentially promote hyperglycemia and/or ß-blockers may potentially interrupt symptoms of hypoglycemia, it is probably most important to achieve blood pressure control, even if these antihypertensive agents are used. Blood pressure control is more important than a theoretical risk of side effects.[88]

C Serious efforts should be made to normalize blood pressure, with frequent reassessment and change in medication if acceptable blood pressures are not being achieved. Over time, polypharmacy is likely to be required to adequately control hypertension in type 2 diabetes.[89]

D Self-management education includes the benefits of blood pressure monitoring and control, target levels, and therapeutic options.

4 Smoking status must be routinely assessed in all patients. Self-management education includes the additional risk of smoking for the person with diabetes, use of alternative nicotine delivery systems, written or video materials, and other resources, including the availability of smoking cessation programs. Generally, if members of the healthcare team demonstrate concern about smoking and its seriousness and display persistence in efforts to help the individual with diabetes to stop smoking, patients are more likely to succeed in this important goal. Even simply asking about smoking in persons with diabetes, if the question is both direct and supportive, can positively impact smoking cessation.

5 In approaching persons with diabetes and dyslipidemia, the following sequence of interventions should be considered:

A Self-management education emphasizing medical nutrition therapy, the benefits of physical activity, limitations in total saturated fat, cholesterol reduction, and meal planning for glycemic control and modest weight loss is essential for patients with lipid abnormalities (see Chapter 1, Medical Nutrition Therapy for Diabetes, and Chapter 2, Exercise, in Diabetes Management Therapies, for more information).

B Optimal glycemic control is sought in concordance with any pharmacologic therapy for dyslipidemia. However, given the findings from recent studies, aggressive lipid reduction treatment is recommended even while glucose control is being pursued.[84,85]

C Pharmacologic treatment includes several classes of lipid-lowering agents for treatment of dyslipidemia. The metabolic effects of some of these agents have been carefully studied as well as their role in preventing adverse macrovascular outcomes. In the past, persons with diabetes have either been excluded from studies or participated in inadequate numbers to make firm judgments about specific agents for persons with diabetes. However, additional studies have been completed and more explicit recommendations now exist.[37,38,90]

- Bile acid binding resins (eg, cholestyramine) are effective but difficult to use over long periods and may increase triglyceride levels.
- Fibric acid derivatives (eg, gemfibrozil) do not alter diabetes control and seem effective in controlling dyslipidemia. Their full effect may not be achieved for several months. These agents are particularly beneficial in controlling elevated triglyceride levels, a common lipid abnormality in poorly controlled type 2 diabetes.
- Nicotinic acid is inexpensive and effective, but past formulations were associated with side effects such as flushing and worsening of glycemic control in type 2 dia-

betes. A recent study of a new formulation of niacin suggests that this medication may be quite effective without these side effects.[91]

- Antioxidant agents that may prevent LDL oxidation are still being evaluated in ongoing coronary prevention trials, although in a recent HOPE study (Heart Outcomes Prevention Evaluation), vitamin E conveyed no benefit.[92]
- Estrogen replacement for women with diabetes is quite logical given the loss of gender protection from atherosclerosis. However, there is still some concern about the effect of estrogens on triglyceride levels. The HERS (Heart and Estrogen/progestin Replacement Study) trial raised concern about the potential harm of hormone replacement therapy in postmenopausal women.[93]
- Subanalyses of recent primary and secondary lipid reduction trials on cardiovascular disease have for the first time allowed some scientific judgment about the benefits of ß-hydroxy-ß-methylglutaryl-coenzyme A (HMG-CoA) reductase inhibitors.[43] It is clear that persons with diabetes experience even a greater benefit from lipid reduction with the statins than persons without diabetes. Thus, even before glycemic control has been achieved, or if it has not been possible to substantially improve glucose regulation, specific antilipid medication should be initiated, probably with the statins.[37,38,94]

D There are now a number of therapeutic pharmacologic agents and educational and nutritional recommendations for most people with diabetes. The challenge is to assist persons with diabetes in managing this increasingly complex regimen. The entire healthcare team must work together to assist patients, considering their individual characteristics, desires, and circumstances.

E Interest in aspirin therapy in the prevention of CVD in persons with diabetes has increased, particularly in view of recent findings that (1) only about 20% of persons with diabetes who should be on aspirin therapy actually take it regularly, and (2) aspirin therapy has important benefits and a low risk of adverse side effects. At present, it is appropriate to prescribe at least 1 baby aspirin per day to persons with diabetes who are at risk for CVD or its progression.[95]

6 For the person with diabetes who experiences an acute myocardial infarction or stroke, many treatment options are now available that were not routinely considered a decade ago. Given the reality that persons with diabetes are not only more likely than persons without diabetes to have a myocardial infarct, die from the infarct, have complications from the heart attack (congestive heart failure), and experience a subsequent myocardial infarct, aggressive interventions at the time a CVD event occurs is warranted (ie, tertiary prevention of CVD).

A The rapid application of thrombolytic therapy is appropriate, with no evidence of greater adverse consequences. Studies have also indicated the benefit of administering an insulin/glucose/potassium solution for both nondiabetic individuals and persons with diabetes.[96] The occurrence of stress hyperglycemia after acute CVD events is highly predictive of poor outcomes.[97] Other agents that should be strongly considered during an acute event are anticoagulants, ACE inhibitors, ß-blockers, nitroglycerine, statins, and aspirin therapy. Acute management of a CVD event should not be different in persons with diabetes and their nondiabetic counterparts.[98,99]

B Recent studies concerning interventions such as angioplasty, bypass grafting, etc, have indicated that coronary artery bypass grafting is preferable in persons with diabetes because of a high 5-year mortality rate among those receiving angio-plasty.[100-103] The diffuse nature of the coronary atherosclerotic lesions in persons with diabetes, as well as the tendency for restenosis, may be so substantial that percutaneous coronary angioplasty is not as effective. Stent replacement, however, does seem to be useful in persons with diabetes.[104]

Key Educational Considerations

1 Explain the significant problems of macrovascular disease in diabetes—the increased susceptibility of patients with diabetes, the synergistic effect of risk factors, which risks are modifiable, and the clinical manifestations of macrovascular disease in diabetes.

2 Inform the person with diabetes and the family of the importance of monitoring the status of lipid and blood pressure control in addition to blood glucose levels. Antilipid and blood pressure medications, and aspirin therapy also should be used. Familiarize the patient with normal and elevated levels of lipids and blood pressure and teach strategies to lower these values.

3 Present the benefits of following a meal plan at the onset of diabetes that is low in saturated fat and contains 5 servings a day of fruits and vegetables, directed at controlling risk factors for CVD.

4 Resources (programs and materials) related to coping skills and modifying cardiovascular risk factors should be explored and made available to patients as appropriate.

5 Nutrition therapy, physical activity, and/or pharmacologic therapy for hyperlipidemia and/or hypertension bring an additional element of complexity to an already challenging preventive treatment program. Thus, health professionals need to recognize patients' efforts and make available needed referrals and resources. Priorities need to be clear to all team members, especially to the person with diabetes and the family. Blood glucose, blood pressure, and lipid goals need to be established by the patient and health-care team.

Self-Review Questions

1 Define macrovascular disease and distinguish it from microvascular complications of diabetes.

2 Explain how macrovascular complications contribute to morbidity and mortality in persons with diabetes.

3 List factors that may contribute to accelerated macrovascular disease in persons with diabetes.

4 Delineate special features of CVD in persons with diabetes, including clinical manifestations, prognosis, and treatment.

5 Describe ways you would assess for the presence of these risk factors in your patients with diabetes and determine the frequency with which assessment should occur.

6 Describe interventional programs that should be initiated to minimize the chance of macrovascular disease developing and/or progressing in persons with diabetes.

Learning Assessment: Case Study

TM, a 46-year-old African-American woman and mother of 3 teenagers, who has a 13-year history of type 2 diabetes, is being seen in your clinic for the first time. She has been treated with insulin (24 units NPH insulin in the morning, 8 units NPH insulin before dinner), but has used no particular meal plan or exercise program. She tests her blood glucose level periodically, usually when she feels bad. She has come to the clinic to be evaluated for shortness of breath with exertion and headaches. Both symptoms have been present for about 2 months but have been increasing in severity over the past 2 weeks. TM has not been routinely followed in any health facility over the past 4 years; she occasionally visits an emergency room for care.

Initial questioning reveals that TM does not adjust her insulin but does take her shots each day. She had a random blood glucose reading of 283 mg/dL (15.7 mmol/L) last week. She urinates frequently, especially at night, and has never had a low blood sugar reaction (she does know what this means). She had been told during a past emergency room visit that she had some high blood pressure, but she was not prescribed any medication and has not had her blood pressure checked in about 2 years. TM has smoked cigarettes for 18 years. She is unaware of any cholesterol, heart, or kidney problems, although she has many family members and relatives with heart disease.

Physical assessment reveals that her blood pressure is 195/108 mm Hg for 2 readings, and she has background diabetic retinopathy, bilateral rales, a heart gallop, 2+ edema, left ventricular hypertrophy by ECG, proteinuria and glucosuria, and a random capillary glucose level of 268 mg/dL (14.9 mmol/L).

Questions for Discussion

1 What general approaches can be used with complex patients such as TM?
2 What would you do first?
3 What would you include in an educational assessment with TM?
4 What approaches can the healthcare team use that demonstrate cultural appropriateness and sensitivity?

Discussion

1 The fact that TM has not been receiving regular evaluation and care is disturbing. However, because she has now come to the clinic when this has not been her pattern over the past 4 years, the healthcare team needs to be particularly sensitive to her presenting concerns. Something must really be bothering her and the healthcare team needs to understand her worries and help her primarily in these areas.

2 Because of the complexity of the case and the fact that TM is new to your clinic, you need to obtain a lot of information during this first visit. This information is essential for appropriate treatment. In addition, depending on the way this information is collected, the process of interacting with her in a sensitive and appropriate way can help establish rapport so that the chances of her returning are enhanced.

3 The concerns of the healthcare team for TM are
   A Her diabetes has not been regularly evaluated and her glucose control is inadequate.
   B She has microvascular (eye) and likely macrovascular (heart) problems, the latter associated with hypertension and tobacco use. Her history and physical findings are strongly suggestive of congestive heart failure.
   C She also may have lipid problems, although this information is not yet known, along with the status of her renal function.

4 Some initial attention to her glycemic and blood pressure status is essential. While it might seem reasonable to admit TM to the hospital to initiate treatment, she indicates that she must return home to care for her family. She also notes that she has only very basic health insurance. The following tasks can be completed at this initial visit:
   A Offer referral to a dietitian for initial meal planning, including some modest efforts at salt restriction, and alter her insulin program to begin to improve her blood glucose control.
   B Start an ACE inhibitor for her hypertension as well as initial treatment of her likely coronary heart failure. An EKG and chest x-ray would help determine whether she has had an acute myocardial event and the extent of her likely heart failure.
   C Establish some mechanisms for follow up at home (ie, call from nurse) before her scheduled return visit. She should also be instructed in daily weight measurement to carefully monitor her CHF. Some baseline laboratory tests for lipid and renal function would also be reasonable.

5 The educator should be concerned with establishing rapport, addressing TM's concerns, and not overwhelming her with too much information at this first visit. Plans for ongoing care and education need to be established with TM. Her clinical picture—particularly her high blood pressure and CHF—may not be acute, but nevertheless requires short-term follow-up. Practical instructions and guidance, such as demonstrating pill taking, should be emphasized.
   A Assess her basic diabetes knowledge, skills, self-management activities, and attitudes as well as her socioeconomic situation and the status of cardiovascular risk factors. Asking about her concerns and why she came to the clinic today will provide information about areas to address during this first visit.
   B Because attention to her blood pressure and blood glucose control is indicated, her monitoring technique should be assessed as well as her ability (including financial) and willingness to do more frequent blood glucose monitoring. The importance of doing daily weights for CHF should also be emphasized. Ask about her interest in smoking cessation to assess her readiness to quit.
   C If she is able to test her blood glucose levels reliably and more frequently, a plan can be developed to determine when to test and how to use the results to improve her glycemic control. A plan for frequent telephone follow-up and a date for returning to your clinic is essential. While her diabetes is certainly of concern, her high blood pressure and cardiac status probably need more immediate attention. Thus, daily weights and possible home monitoring of blood pressure should be considered.

6 Part of the reason that TM may not have sought health care may be related to past negative experiences with the healthcare system. It is therefore important to address

TM by her last name, treat her with respect, and avoid making judgments about her self-care behaviors and lack of past medical care. It is also important to assess her cultural and religious beliefs and practices that may influence the way she cares for her diabetes. Incorporate ethnic foods into her meal plan as appropriate, and ask about her use of alternative therapies.

References

1 Zimmet P. Globalization, coca-colonization and the chronic disease epidemic: can the Doomsday scenario be averted. J Intern Med. 2000;247:301-310.

2 King H, Aubert R, Herman W. Global burden of diabetes, 1995-2025: prevalence, numerical estimates and projections. Diabetes Care. 1998;21:1414-1431.

3 Mokdad A, Ford E, Bowman B, et al. Diabetes trends in the US: 1990-1998. Diabetes Care. 2000;23:1278-1283.

4 Fagot-Campagna A, Pettit D, Engelgau M, et al. Type 2 diabetes among North American children and adolescents: an epidemiologic review and a public health perspective. J Pediatr. 2000;136:664-672.

5 Beckles G, Engelgau M, Narayan K, et al. Population-based assessment of the level of care among adults with diabetes in the US. Diabetes Care. 1998; 21:1432-1438.

6 Mann J. Stemming the tide of diabetes mellitus. Lancet. 2000;356:1454-1455.

7 Hodgson T, Cohen A. Medical care expenditures for diabetes, its chronic complications, and its co-morbidities. Prev Med. 1999;29:173-186.

8 Keen H, Clark C, Laakso M. Reducing the burden of diabetes: managing cardiovascular disease. Diabetes Metab Res Rev. 1999;15:186-196.

9 McGuire D, Granger C. Diabetes and ischemic heart disease. Am Heart J. 1999;138:S366-S375.

10 Nash D. Diabetes mellitus and cardiovascular disease. Diabetes Educ. 2001;27:28-34.

11 American Diabetes Association. Economic consequences of diabetes mellitus in the US in 1997. Diabetes Care. 1998;21:296-309.

12 Newby A, Libby P, van der Wal A. Plaque instability: the real challenge for atherosclerosis research in the next decade? Cardiovasc Res. 1999;41:321-322.

13 Rauch U, Osende J, Fuster V, et al. Thrombus formation on atherosclerotic plaques: pathogenesis and clinical consequences. Ann Intern Med. 2001;134:224-238.

14 Kullo I, Edwards W, Schwartz R. Vulnerable plaque: pathobiology and clinical implications. Ann Intern Med. 1998;129:1050-1060.

15 Libby P. Changing concepts of atherogenesis. J Intern Med. 2000;247:349-358.

16 Welty F. Cardiovascular disease and dyslipidemia in women. Arch Intern Med. 2001;161:514-522.

17 Steinberg H, Paradisi G, Cronin J, et al. Type 2 diabetes abrogates sex differences in endothelial function in premenopausal women. Circulation. 2000;101:2040-2046.

18 Grundy S, Benjamin I, Burke G, et al. Diabetes and cardiovascular disease: a statement for healthcare professionals from the American Heart Association. Circulation. 1999;100:1134-1146.

19 Miettinen H, Lehto S, Salomaa V, et al. Impact of diabetes on mortality after the first myocardial infarction. The FIN-MONICA Myocardial Infarction Register Study Group. Diabetes Care. 1998;21:69-75.

20 Lotufo P, Gaziano J, Chae C, et al. Diabetes and all-cause and coronary heart disease mortality among US male physicians. Arch Intern Med. 2001;161:242-247.

21 Fonesca V. Risk factors for coronary heart disease in diabetes. Ann Intern Med. 2000;135:154-156.

22 Vinicor F. Features of macrovascular disease of diabetes. In: Haire-Joshu D, ed. Management of Diabetes Mellitus: Perspectives of Care Across the Life Span. 2nd ed. St. Louis: Mosby-Year Book Inc; 1996:281-308.

23 Benson R, Sacco R. Stroke prevention: hypertension, diabetes, tobacco, and lipids. Neurol Clin. 2000;18:309-319.

24 Haffner S, Lehto S, Ronnemaa T, et al. Mortality from coronary heart disease in subjects with type 2 diabetes and in nondiabetic subjects with and without prior myocardial infarction. N Engl J Med. 1998;339:229-234.

25 Mortality from coronary heart disease and acute myocardial infarction—United States: 1998. MMWR. 2001;50:90-93.

26 Gu K, Cowie C, Harris M. Diabetes and decline in heart disease mortality in US adults. JAMA. 1999;281:1291-1297.

27 Haffner S. Coronary heart disease in patients with diabetes. N Engl J Med. 2000;342:1040-1042.

28 Kloner R. Cardiovascular risk and sildenafil. Am J Cardiol. 2000;86:57F-61F.

29 Perry R, Baron A. Impaired glucose tolerance: why is it not a disease? Diabetes Care. 1999; 22:883-885.

30 Mankovsky B, Metzer B, Molitch M, et al. Cerebrovascular disorders in patients with diabetes mellitus. J Diabetes Complications. 1996;10:228-242.

31 Ollendorf D, Kotsanos J, Wishner W, et al. Potential economic benefits of lower-extremity amputation prevention strategies in diabetes. Diabetes Care. 1998;21:1240-1245.

32 Centers for Disease Control. Diabetes Surveillance, 1999. Available at: http://www.cdc.gov/diabetes/statistics/index.htm. Accessed April 2001.

33 Clark C, Perry R. Type 2 diabetes and macrovascular disease: epidemiology and etiology. Am Heart J. 1999;138:S330-S333.

34 Will J, Vinicor F, Stevenson J. Recording of diabetes on death certificates: has it improved? J Clin Epidemiol. 2001;54:239-244.

35 Eastman R, Keen H. The impact of cardiovascular disease in people with diabetes: the potential for prevention. Lancet. 1997;350:S129-S132.

36 Yudkin J, Chaturvedi N. Developing risk stratification charts for diabetic and non-diabetic subjects. Diabetic Med. 1999;16:219-227.

37 Haffner SM. Management of dyslipidemia in adults with diabetes (technical review). Diabetes Care. 1998;21:160-178.

38 American Diabetes Association. Management of dyslipidemia in adults with diabetes (position statement). Diabetes Care. 2001;24:S58-S61.

39 Stewart M, Heiss G, Cohn R, et al. Triglycerides in diabetes: time for action? Diabetic Med. 1994;11:725-727.

40 Haffner S. Secondary prevention of coronary heart disease: the role of fibric acids. Circulation. 2000;102:2-4.

41 Ceriello A. The post-prandial state and cardiovascular disease: relevance to diabetes mellitus. Diabetes Metab Res Rev. 2000;16:125-132.

42 Haffner S. The importance of hyperglycemia in the nonfasting state to the development of cardiovascular disease. Endocrinol Rev. 1998;19:583-592.

43 Calles-Escandon J, Cipolla M. Diabetes and endothelial dysfunction: a clinical perspective. Endocrinol Rev. 2001;22:36-52.

44 Haffner SM, Stern MP, Hazuda HP, Mitchell BD, Patterson JK. Cardiovascular risk factors in confirmed pre-diabetic individuals. Does the clock for coronary heart disease start ticking before the onset of clinical diabetes? JAMA. 1990;263:2893-2898.

45 Haffner S. Do interventions to reduce coronary heart disease reduce the incidence of type 2 diabetes? A possible role for inflammatory factors. Circulation. 2001;103:346-351.

46 Festa A, D'Agostino R, Howard G, et al. Chronic subclinical inflammation as part of the insulin resistance syndrome: the Insulin Resistance Atherosclerosis Study (IRAS). Circulation. 2000;102:42-47.

47 Adler A, Stratton I, Neil H, et al. Association of systolic blood pressure with macrovascular and microvascular complications of type 2 diabetes (UKPDS 36): prospective observational study. BMJ. 2000;321:412-419.

48 Hansson L, Zanchetti A, Carruthers S, et al. Effects of intensive blood-pressure lowering and low-dose aspirin in patients with hypertension: principal results of the Hypertension Optimal Treatment (HOT) randomized trial. Lancet. 1998;351:1755-1762.

49 Heart Outcome Prevention Evaluation Study Investigators. Effects of ramipril on cardiovascular and microvascular outcomes in people with diabetes mellitus: results of the HOPE and MICRO-HOPE substudy. Lancet. 2000;355:253-259.

50 McGuire D. Influence of proteinuria on long-term outcome among patients with diabetes: the evidence continues to accumulate. Am Heart J. 2000;139:934-935.

51 McFarlane S, Banerji M, Sowers J. Insulin resistance and cardiovascular disease. J Clin Endocrinol Metab. 2001;86:713-718.

52 Khaw K, Wareham N, Luben R, et al. Glycated haemoglobin, diabetes and mortality in men in Norfolk cohort of European Prospective Investigation of Cancer and Nutrition. BMJ. 2001;322:15-18.

53 Barrett-Conner E, Wingrad D. "Normal" blood glucose and coronary risk: dose response effects seem consistent throughout the glycaemic continuum. BMJ. 2001;322:5-6.

54 Godfrey K, Barker D. Fetal nutrition and adult disease. Am J Clin Nutr. 2000;71(S5):1344-1352.

55 Ravelli A, van der Meulen J, Osmond C, et al. Infant feeding and adult glucose tolerance, lipid profile, blood pressure and obesity. Arch Dis Child. 2000;82:248-252.

56 Haire-Joshu D, Glasgow R, Tibbs T. Smoking and diabetes (technical review). Diabetes Care. 1999;22:1887-1898.

57 Will J, Ford E, Galuska D, Calle E. Diabetes, a consequence of smoking? Int J Epidemiol. 2001. In press.

58 Nakanishi N, Nakamura K, Matsuo Y, et al. Cigarette smoking and risk for impaired fasting glucose and type 2 diabetes: in middle-aged Japanese men. Ann Intern Med. 2000;133:183-192.

59 Vlassara H. Advanced glycation end products and atherosclerosis. Ann Med. 1996;28:419-426.

60 Hu F, Stampfer M, Solomon C, et al. Physical activity and risk for cardiovascular events in diabetic women. Ann Intern Med. 2001;134:96-105.

61 Rodgers G, Ayanian J, Balady G, et al. A report of the American College of Cardiology/American Heart Association/American College of Physicians. American Society of Internal Medicine Task Force on Clinical Competence statement on stress testing. J Am Coll Cardiol. 2000;36:1441-1453.

62 Adler A, Turner R. The diabetes prevention program. Diabetes Care. 1999;22:543-545.

63 Liu S, Willett W, Stampfer M, et al. A prospective study of dietary glycemic load, carbohydrate intake, and risk of coronary heart disease in US women. Am J Clin Nutr. 2000;71:1455-1461.

64 Ajani W, Gaziano J, Lotufo P, et al. Alcohol consumption and risk of coronary heart disease by diabetes status. Circulation. 2000;102:500-505.

65 Colwell J. Aspirin therapy in diabetes (technical review). Diabetes Care. 1997;20:1767-1771.

66 Rolka D, Fagot-Campagna A, Narayan K. Aspirin use among adults with diabetes: estimates from the Third National Health and Nutritional Examination Survey. Diabetes Care. 2001; 24:197-201.

67 UKPDS Group. Intensive blood-glucose control with sulfonylurea or insulin compared with conventional treatment and risk of complications in patients with type 2 diabetes (UKPDS 32). Lancet. 1998;352:837-853.

68 Reaven G. Insulin resistance: a chicken that has come to roost. Ann New York Acad Sci. 1999;892:45-57.

69 Adler A, Neil H, Manley S, et al. Hyperglycemia and hyperinsulinemia at diagnosis of diabetes and their association with subsequent cardiovascular disease in the United Kingdom Prospective Diabetes Study (UKPDS 47). Am Heart J. 1999;138:353-359.

70 Bakris G, Sowers J, Epstein M, et al. Hypertension in patients with diabetes. Why is aggressive treatment essential? Postgrad Med. 2000;107:53-56.

71 Fuller J, Stevens L, Chaturvedi, et al. Antihypertensive therapy for preventing cardiovascular complications in people with diabetes mellitus. Cochrane Database Systematic Rev. 2000;(2):CD002188.

72 Fries E. Improving treatment effectiveness in hypertension. Arch Intern Med. 1999;159:2517-2521.

73 Nishikawa T, Edelstein D, Du X, et al. Normalizing mitochondria superoxide production blocks three pathways of hyperglycaemic damage. Nature. 2000;404: 787-790.

74 Haffner S. Epidemiological studies on the effects of hyperglycemia and improvement of glycemic control on macrovascular events in type 2 diabetes. Diabetes Care. 1999; 22:54-56.

75 Wild S, Dunn C, McKeigue P, et al. Glycemic control and cardiovascular disease in type 2 diabetes: a review. Diabetes Metab Res Rev. 1999;15:197-204.

76 Diabetes Control and Complications Trial Research Group. The effect of intensive treatment of diabetes on the development and progression of long-term complications of insulin-dependent diabetes. N Engl J Med. 1993;329:977-986.

77 Ohkubo Y, Kishikawa H, Araki E, et al. Intensive insulin therapy prevents the progression of diabetic microvascular complications in Japanese patients with non-insulin dependent diabetes mellitus: a randomized prospective 6-year study. Diabetes Res Clin Pract. 1995;18:103-117.

78 Abraira C, McGuire D. Intensive insulin therapy in patients with type 2 diabetes: implications of the Veterans Affairs (VA CSDM) feasibility trial. Am Heart J. 138: S360-S365.

79 Colwell J. Elevated plasma homocysteine and diabetic vascular disease. Diabetes Care. 1997;20:1805-1806.

80 Eikelboom J, Lann E, Genest J, et al. Homocysteine and cardiovascular disease: a critical review of the epidemiologic evidence. Ann Intern Med. 1999;131:363-375.

81 Stephens M. Is electron-beam computed tomography (EBCT) a reliable tool for predicting coronary outcomes in an asymptomatic population? J Fam Pract. 2000; 49:688.

82 Haffner S. Is all coronary heart disease prevention in type 2 diabetes mellitus secondary prevention? J Clin Endocrinol Metab. 2000;85:2108-2110.

83 Haffner S. Management of dyslipidemia in adults with diabetes (technical review). Diabetes Care. 1998;21:160-178.

84 Gover S, Coupal L, Zowall H, et al. Cost-effectiveness of treating hyperlipidemia in the presence of diabetes: who should be treated? Circulation. 2000;102;722-727.

85 Deedwania P. Hypertension and diabetes: new therapeutic options. Arch Intern Med. 2000;160:1585-1594.

86 Peters A, Hsueh W. Antihypertensive agents in diabetic patients: great benefits, special risks. Arch Intern Med. 1999;159:541-542.

87 Elliot W, Weir D, Black H. Cost-effectiveness of the lower treatment goal (of JNC VI) for diabetic hypertensive patients. Joint National Committee on Prevention, Detection, Evaluation and Treatment of High Blood Pressure. Arch Intern Med. 2000;160:1277-1288.

88 Joint National Committee on Prevention, Detection, Evaluation and Treatment of High Blood Pressure. The sixth report of the Joint National Committee on prevention and treatment of high blood pressure. Arch Intern Med. 1997;157:2413-2446.

89 Turner R, Cull C, Frighi V, et al. Glycemic control with diet, sulfonylurea, metformin, or insulin in patients with type 2 diabetes mellitus: progressive requirement for multiple therapies (UKPDS 49). JAMA. 1999;281:2005-2012.

90 Ballantyne C, Grundy S, Oberman A, et al. Hyperlipidemia: diagnostic and therapeutic perspectives. J Clin Endocrinol Metab. 2000;85:2089-2112.

91 Wolfe M, Vartanian S, Ross J, et al. Safety and effectiveness of Niaspan when added sequentially to a statin for treatment of dyslipidemia. Am J Cardiol. 2001;87:476-479.

92 Hoogwerf B, Young J. The HOPE study. Ramipril lowered cardiovascular risk, but vitamin E did not. Clev Clin J Med. 2000;67:287-293.

93 Hulley S, Drady D, Bush T, et al. Randomized trial of estrogen plus progestin for secondary prevention of coronary heart disease in postmenopausal women. Heart and Estrogen/progestin Replacement (HERS) Research Group. JAMA. 1998;280:605-613.

94 Kreisberg R. Diabetic dyslipidemia. Am J Cardiol. 1998;82(12A):67-73,85-86.

95 Colwell J. Aspirin therapy in diabetes is underutilized. Diabetes Care. 2001;24:195-196.

96 Malmberg K, McGuire D. Diabetes and acute myocardial infarction: the role of insulin therapy. Am Heart J. 1999;138:S381-S386.

97 Capes S, Hunt D, Malmberg K, et al. Stress hyperglycemia and increased risk of death after myocardial infarction in patients with and without diabetes: a systematic overview. Lancet. 2000;355:773-778.

98 Mak K, Topol E. Emerging concepts in the management of acute myocardial infarction in patients with diabetes mellitus. J Am Coll Cardiol. 2000;35:563-568.

99 Friesinger C, Gavin J. Diabetes and the cardiologists: a call to action. J Am Coll Cardiol. 2000;35:1130-1133.

100 King S. Coronary artery bypass graft or percutaneous coronary interventions in patients with diabetes: another nail in the coffin or "too close to call?" J Am Coll Cardiol. 2001;37:1016-1018.

101 Niles N, McGrath P, Malenka D, et al. Survival of patients with diabetes and multivessel coronary artery disease after surgical or percutaneous coronary revascularization: results of a large regional prospective study. J Am Coll Cardiol. 2001; 37:1008-1015.

102 The Bypass Angioplasty Revascularization Investigation (BARI) Investigators. Comparison of coronary bypass surgery with angioplasty in patients with multivessel disease. N Engl J Med. 1996;335:217-225.

103 Sobel B. Acceleration of restenosis by diabetes: pathogenetic implications. Circulation. 2001;103:1185-1187.

104 Lincoff A. Potent complementary clinical benefit of abciximab and stenting during percutaneous coronary revascularization in patients with diabetes mellitus: results of the EPISTENT trial. Am Heart J. 2000;139:S46-S52.

Suggested Readings

American Diabetes Association. Detection and management of lipid disorders in diabetes (consensus statement). Diabetes Care. 1993;16:828-834.

Atherosclerosis and diabetes. Diabetes Rev. 1997;5(4).

Colwell JA. Aspirin therapy in diabetes (technical review). Diabetes Care. 1997;20:1767-1771.

Diabetes and arteriosclerosis. Int Diabetes Fed Bull. 1997;(Nov):V 42.

Haffner SM. Management of dyslipidemia in adults with diabetes (technical review). Diabetes Care. 1998;21:160-178.

Haire-Joshu D, Glasgow RE, Tibbs TL. Smoking and diabetes (technical review). Diabetes Care. 1999;22:1887-1898.

Hansson L, Zanchetti S, Carruthers G, et al, for the HOT Study Group. Effects of intensive blood-pressure lowering and low-dose aspirin in patients with hypertension: principal results of the Hypertension Optimal Treatment (HOT) randomized trial. Lancet. 1998; 351:1755-1782.

Herman WH, Alexander CN, Cook JR, et al. Effect of simvastatin treatment on cardiovascular resource utilization in impaired fasting glucose and diabetes: findings from the Scandinavian Simvastatin Survival Study. Diabetes Care. 1999;22:1771-1778.

Stratton IM, Adler AI, Neil HA, et al. Association of glycaemia with macrovascular and microvascular complications of type 2 diabetes (UKPDS 35): prospective observational study. BMJ. 2000;321:1405-1412.

Turner RC, Millns H, Neil HA, et al. Risk factors for coronary artery disease in non-insulin-dependent diabetes mellitus (UKPDS 23). BMJ. 1998;316:823-828.

Learning Assessment: Post-Test Questions

Macrovascular Disease   6

1   Fifty to sixty percent of all deaths in persons with diabetes can be attributed to:
  A Microvascular disease
  B Coronary artery disease
  C Peripheral vascular disease
  D Cerebral vascular disease

2   What impact does diabetes have on the development of coronary artery disease in women compared with men?
  A Women have a higher risk than men
  B Men have a higher risk than women
  C The risk is minimal in both sexes
  D The risk is the same for both sexes

3   Which of the following is not a usual symptom of acute coronary insufficiency?
  A Angina
  B Flushing
  C Diaphoresis
  D Anxiety

4   Improved glycemic control does which of the following?
  A Decreases triglycerides and increases HDL
  B Increases plasma fibrinogen levels
  C Increases HDL levels independent of changes in lipid levels
  D Has little effect on platelet behavior

5   The presence of hypertension in persons with type 1 diabetes is correlated with:
  A Weight and insulin resistance
  B Duration of diabetes and renal function
  C Low HDL levels and physical inactivity
  D Presence of AGEs and elevated glucose levels

6   Which of the following medications should be used with caution when treating hypertension in persons with diabetes?
  A ß-blockers
  B Angiotensin converting enzyme inhibitors
  C Statins
  D Aspirin therapy

7   Which of the following statements is the least accurate about peripheral vascular disease (PVD)?
  A Absent peripheral pulses occur with approximately the same frequency in persons with type 1 and type 2 diabetes
  B Patient education efforts should emphasize foot care
  C People with diabetes have a 15 times higher age-related risk for amputation
  D PVD is clinically characterized by intermittent claudication and foot ulcers

8   The elements that commonly characterize the metabolic syndrome are:
  A Hyperglycemia, central obesity, neuropathy, and microalbuminuria
  B Hyperglycemia, hyperlipidemia, hypertension, and central obesity
  C Hyperlipidemia, hypertension, and family history of cardiovascular disease
  D Hypoglycemia, neuropathy, hyperinsulinemia, and pregnancy

9   In the development of cardiovascular disease, smoking is associated with:
  A Elevated HDL levels
  B Decreased fibrinogen levels
  C Development of advanced glycosylated end products (AGEs)
  D Formation of stable plaques with a thick fibrous cap

10   JS is a 45-year-old female patient with type 2 diabetes. Her blood pressure is 170/95. She has elevated LDL cholesterol and total cholesterol. Her fasting blood glucose level is 130 mg/dL. What additional information would be most helpful to complete your assessment and develop an intervention strategy for her cardiovascular complications?
  A Food habits
  B Age at time diabetes was first diagnosed
  C Ethnicity and family history of cardiovascular disease
  D Use of antihypertensive agents

See next page for answer key.

Post-Test Answer Key

Macrovascular Disease   6

1	B		6	A
2	D		7	A
3	B		8	B
4	A		9	C
5	B		10	A

Eye Disease and Adaptive Diabetes Education for Visually Impaired Persons

Marla Bernbaum, MD
St. Louis University Health Sciences Center
Division of Endocrinology
St. Louis, Missouri

Tamara Stich, RN, MSN, CDE
Washington University School of Medicine
Department of Metabolism
St. Louis, Missouri

Introduction

1 Diabetes is a leading cause of vision impairment in the United States. Diabetic retinopathy is the most prevalent ophthalmic disease among individuals with diabetes. However, persons with diabetes are also at increased risk for other eye conditions that may impact visual function. Those who acquire impaired vision during the course of their diabetes, as well as persons with preexisting vision loss due to other causes, need adaptive skills for diabetes self-management.

2 The extent of vision impairment and the individual's ability to adapt to the vision loss must be evaluated before undertaking adaptive education. The adaptive education and training needs of persons with preexisting eye disease due to other causes may differ from persons experiencing a new onset of diabetic retinopathy.

3 The diabetes educator can play a key role in referring patients with visual impairment to the proper rehabilitative and psychosocial services.

4 This chapter provides basic information regarding risk factors, screening, and treatment for diabetic eye disease and describes skills required for working with visually impaired patients with diabetes.

Objectives

Upon completion of this chapter, the learner will be able to

1 Describe the stages of diabetic retinopathy and appropriate treatment for each stage.

2 List 6 other ophthalmic conditions that may occur more commonly in people with diabetes than in the general population.

3 Identify 3 factors for assessing function with vision loss.

4 Identify the appropriate time for referral and the general services that are available for individuals with diabetes and visual impairment.

5 List 5 ways to enhance interactions with individuals who are visually impaired.

6 Describe 5 ways to adapt diabetes self-management skills for the visually impaired patient.

Identifying and Treating Diabetic Eye Disease

1 Diabetes is the leading cause of blindness in the United States for persons between the ages of 20 and 74 years.[1-6]

  A Eye disease is 25 times more common among people with diabetes than in the general population.[4]

    • Diabetes accounts for 12% of legal blindness in the US.[2,3]

    • Literature suggests there are 8 000 to 23 000 new cases of legal blindness associated with diabetes annually.[1-6]

    • Incidence and prevalence rates for less severe levels of vision impairment are not established, although prevalence of significant vision loss among persons with diabetes appears to exceed 570 000 and may extend well above 1 million.[6]

  B Persons with both type 1 and type 2 diabetes are susceptible to diabetic retinopathy, the most prevalent diabetic eye complication.

- Diabetic retinopathy is often detectable within 5 years of the diagnosis of diabetes.[2,4,5]
- Since type 2 diabetes may go undetected for well over 5 years after the onset, 21% of type 2 patients already have retinopathy at the time of diagnosis.
- Twenty years after the diagnosis of diabetes, more than 90% of persons acquiring the disease at less than 30 years of age develop nonproliferative retinopathy; 50% progress to proliferative retinopathy. (Onset at less than or greater than 30 years implies, in this case, type 1 or type 2 diabetes.)
- After 20 years, nonproliferative retinopathy is present in 80% of persons over age 30 at onset of diabetes who are treated with insulin and in 20% of those who do not require insulin treatment; 40% and 5%, respectively, progress to proliferative retinopathy.
- Risk for clinically significant macular edema is 10% to 15% for all persons having diabetes for 15 to 20 or more years.
- Over 600 000 persons are in the stage of the disease at which vision is threatened (ie, high-risk proliferative disease or clinically significant macular edema). (Table 7.1).

Table 7.1. Percentage of Persons With Diabetic Retinopathy 20 Years After Diagnosis of Diabetes[4]

Stage of Retinopathy	Age of Onset and Type of Diabetes		
	Age <30, Type 1	Age ≥30, Treated With Insulin	Age ≥30, Treated Without Insulin
Retinopathy All Stages	>90%	80%	20%
Proliferative	50%	40%	5%
Clinically significant macular edema	10%-15% all groups		

C One half to two thirds of the approximately 30% of persons with diabetes who are on work disability have vision impairment.[1,4,5,7]
- The financial impact in terms of Social Security and disability benefits is estimated at $6900 per person annually.
- The cost of the recommended treatment is estimated at $2000 per person per year of vision spared.
- Only 60% of people with diabetes receive needed ophthalmologic treatment.
- Greater than 90% of vision loss could be prevented by appropriate therapy.

D The development and progression of retinopathy correlates strongly with degree of glycemic control in addition to duration of diabetes.[3-5]
- This relationship was demonstrated in the Diabetes Control and Complications Trial (DCCT) and the United Kingdom Prospective Diabetes Study (UKPDS);[8,9] the results emphasized the importance of achieving the best possible glucose control in all persons with diabetes.

- Other risk factors for diabetic retinopathy include age, hypertension, hyperlipidemia, smoking, and genetic predisposition.[10,11]
- Puberty, pregnancy, and renal failure can potentiate retinopathy.
- Retinopathy is rarely detected prior to onset of puberty.

2 Diabetic retinopathy[3-5,12,13] occurs when the microvasculature that nourishes the retina is damaged, permitting leakage of blood components through the vessel walls. The retina is a layer of nerve tissue at the back of the eye that is responsible for focusing images and light, which then are relayed along the optic nerve to the brain (Figure 7.1). Retinopathy may vary from a mild asymptomatic form to a severe, rapidly devastating condition. Retinopathy is staged from its mildest to most advanced form using the terms nonproliferative (mild, moderate, severe, and very severe) and proliferative retinopathy. (Note: the terms background retinopathy and preproliferative retinopathy are no longer considered current.)[4,5] (See Table 7.2.)

A Retinopathy before the development of retinal neovascularization is termed *nonproliferative diabetic retinopathy* (NPDR). Mild NPDR often causes no visual disturbance. It may remain asymptomatic for years, and the following specific features may be noted on ophthalmoscopic exam:[4,5]

- *Microaneurysms* are seen as sacular outpouchings along weakened vascular walls.
- *Hard exudates*, the residue of fluid and lipid components that leak from the blood vessels, appear as round, yellow deposits on the retina.
- *Intraretinal hemorrhages* may appear as dots or flame shapes.
- *Cotton-wool spots* or soft exudates represent infarcts of the nerve fiber layer of the retina.

B As the disease progresses, there is evidence of further vascular damage, capillary obstruction or closure, and retinal ischemia. Persons with very severe NPDR have a 45% risk of proliferative changes within 1 year but may not experience detectable vision impairment. Moderate-to-very severe nonproliferative retinopathy is staged according to the extent of the following characteristics: [4,5]

- *Intraretinal hemorrhages* that are more extensive in both size and number.
- *Venous beading* appears as changes in the appearance of the retinal veins as they become tortuous and swollen, loop back upon themselves, and take on the appearance of a string of sausages or beads.
- *Intraretinal microvascular abnormalities* (IRMA) appear as dilated capillaries that arise around ischemic areas where there is capillary closure.

C Once proliferation of new retinal vessels occurs, it is referred to as *proliferative diabetic retinopathy* (PDR). PDR is thought to develop as a result of retinal ischemia and hypoxia following capillary closure. Proliferative changes, the process of *neovascularization*, is defined as the growth of new blood vessels along the surface of the retina; these vessels may extend into the vitreous chamber using the vitreous surface as a scaffold. The vessels are fragile and rupture easily, producing preretinal and vitreous hemorrhage. The resulting vision impairment may vary from mild blurring with cobweb-like wisps in the visual fields to severe obstruction of vision due to large, dense opacities.

- *Neovascularization of the disk* (NVD) refers to new vessel growth on or near the optic disk as opposed to neovascularization elsewhere on the retina (NVE). Preretinal or vitreous hemorrhage in combination with NVD or NVD alone that is greater than 25% of the surface area of the disk are considered high-risk features for major vision loss.

Figure 7.1. Normal Eye

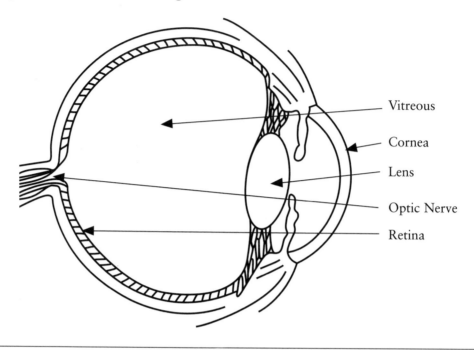

Vitreous

Cornea

Lens

Optic Nerve

Retina

Source: Reprinted with permission from Noninsulin-Dependent Diabetes Mellitus: a curriculum for patients and health professionals, Michigan Diabetes Research and Training Center, The University of Michigan, 1988.

Table 7.2. Stages of Diabetic Retinopathy

Early Stages *Mild NPDR*	• Retinal vascular microaneurysms and blot hemorrhages • Increased retinal vascular permeability • Cotton wool spots
Middle Stages *Moderate NPDR* *Severe NPDR* *Very Severe NPDR*	• Venous caliber changes or beading • IRMA • Retinal capillary loss • Retinal ischemia • Extensive intraretinal hemorrhages and microaneurysms
Advanced Stages *PDR*	• NVD • NVE • Neovascularization of the iris • Neovascular glaucoma • Preretinal and vitreous hemorrhage • Fibrovascular proliferation • Retinal traction, retinal tears, retinal detachment

Source: Reprinted with permission from Aiello LP, Gardner TW, King GL, et al.[5]

- Another potential threat to vision results as fibrous components of the neovasculature contract, leading to retinal traction, detachments, and tears.

D *Macular edema* is a serious consequence of leakage of fluid and exudate from the vessels in the macula, which is the specialized portion of the retina responsible for central vision.[4,5]

- Macular edema may accompany nonproliferative or proliferative retinopathy.
- *Clinically significant macular edema* (CSME) is established when resulting retinal thickening and exudates are sufficient to threaten or impair the central vision.
- Vision loss may vary from mild blurring to an acuity of 20/200 or less (legal blindness).
- Clinically significant macular edema, which requires early treatment, is assessed by slitlamp biomicroscopy and stereoscopic fundus photography; fluorescein angiography is used to guide treatment and to monitor progression and therapeutic results.

E Neovascular glaucoma and neovascularization of the iris (rubeosis iridis) are relatively rare complications associated with proliferative retinopathy.[5]

- New vessels proliferate from the surface of the iris, blocking aqueous outflow from the anterior chamber of the eye.
- The condition is painful, progresses rapidly, and is devastating to vision.

3 Treatment of retinopathy begins with preventive measures such as optimizing blood glucose, lipids and blood pressure, and smoking cessation. Routine annual screening and follow-up by an ophthalmologist are essential to assure that any intervention is appropriately timed.[4,5,12-16]

A Mild-to-moderate nonproliferative retinopathy requires only observation.

B Severe-to-very severe nonproliferative retinopathy is not treated in type 1 patients. However, panretinal photocoagulation may be applied in persons with type 2 diabetes, for whom benefits to vision have been shown to outweigh risks of the therapy.[13]

- Stereoscopic color fundus photography and slitlamp biomicroscopy may be recommended for persons with NPDR to document stage and progression of retinopathy and to detect macular edema and/or macular ischemia.

C Macular edema which is not clinically significant is observed, but not treated.

D Clinically significant macular edema is treated with focal argon photocoagulation to seal leaking blood vessels. Multiple applications are often necessary. Early treatment reduces vision loss by 50% after 3 years.[14]

- Fluorescein angiography is used to guide treatment of CSME and to monitor progression and therapeutic response, but generally is not indicated for assessing other categories of retinopathy (where benefit does not justify associated discomfort and risk for allergic reaction).

E Proliferative retinopathy with high-risk characteristics should be treated with panretinal photocoagulation in which laser treatments are applied to the peripheral retina in a scatter pattern.[15] Severe vision loss is reduced by 60% to 90% after 3 years.

- Side effects of therapy may include a small loss of visual acuity (about 1 line on the Snellen chart) as well as some decrement in peripheral vision, dark adaptation, and color discrimination. These effects should be offset by preservation of the central vision.
- Type 1 patients with less than high-risk PDR do not gain sufficient benefits to justify visual risks associated with treatment.

- Patients with type 2 diabetes who have less than high-risk proliferative characteristics do gain net benefit from photocoagulation.[13]
- Advise patients that multiple treatment sessions are often necessary and there may be mild eye discomfort. For patients with severe pain, a local anesthetic injection to the eye may be used, although most patients require only anesthetic eye drops.
- Treatment is performed on an outpatient basis. Patients can return to normal activities the next day.

F Surgical vitrectomy is considered for hemorrhages that do not resolve over 6 months or when there is a threatened or actual retinal detachment.[16] An ultrasound may be used to detect detachments when there is dense vitreous hemorrhage.
- The vitreous contents, including hemorrhage and fibrous proliferation, are removed and replaced by a clear solution. Repair of the retina may be undertaken during the procedure.
- Surgical complications such as corneal edema, retinal tears, recurrent hemorrhage, and rubeosis may be as high as 25%.[4] The risks and benefits should be carefully explored with the patient.

G Panretinal photocoagulation may be of benefit in neovascular glaucoma prior to attempting surgical filtration procedures. Cryotherapy also may be helpful.

H An important aspect of treatment is meeting the patient's needs in adapting to loss of vision.[17-21]
- Offer psychosocial counseling before there is actual deterioration of vision to help allay anxiety and depression.
- Low-vision evaluation is indicated as soon as vision loss impacts normal daily activities.
- Referral to rehabilitation services as early as possible will allow the patient to acquire adaptive skills and maintain participation and independence in work and recreational activities.
- Patients need information and instruction in adaptive diabetes self-care as soon as vision is compromised, preferably before adaptive equipment is actually required.

4 Other ocular complications are associated with diabetes.[2,12,22]
  A Common senile cataracts occur more frequently, at younger ages, and progress more rapidly in persons with diabetes.
  B The diabetic cataract is a rare type of cataract associated with osmotic irregularity that can mature in a few days and progress very rapidly.
  C There is increased risk of primary open-angled glaucoma, the most common kind of glaucoma in the US.
  D Ischemic optic neuropathy refers to irreversible optic nerve damage due to microvascular impairment. This ocular complication occurs more frequently in persons with diabetes and leads to permanent visual impairment.
  E Ocular palsies result from ischemia to the third, fourth, and sixth cranial nerves. Impairment of extraocular muscle function leads to strabismus or diplopia. This can occur as a kind of diabetic neuropathy. The condition is temporary and normal function usually returns within a few months.
  F Blurring of vision due to instability of blood glucose is related to osmotic changes in the lens of the eye. This problem occurs commonly at the onset of diabetes and

during periods of fluctuating control. Reassure the patient that this condition is transient. Instruct patients to delay testing for new refractive lenses until the blood glucose has been stabilized for 6 to 8 weeks.

G Temporary visual changes such as dimming of vision, bright flashing lights, or double vision may be experienced during periods of hypoglycemia.

5 All persons with diabetes should receive routine ophthalmologic screening and follow-up. Indirect ophthalmoscopy with slitlamp examination and measurement of the intraocular pressure are essential.[4,5,23]

A A dilated examination is recommended annually beginning 3 to 5 years after the diagnosis of diabetes for patients who are age 10 to 29 and annually beginning at the time of diagnosis for patients 30 years and older.

B Since pregnancy potentiates retinopathy, women should have an examination during preconception planning, the first trimester of pregnancy, and close follow-up as needed.

C If retinopathy is identified, fundus photography or fluorescein angiography may be recommended, and more frequent eye examinations are needed (Table 7.3).

Table 7.3. Schedule for Ophthalmologic Examination

Stage of Retinopathy	Frequency of Examination
No retinopathy	Annually
Mild nonproliferative retinopathy	Annually
Moderate nonproliferative retinopathy/macular edema	6 to 12 months
Clinically significant macular edema or severe-to-very severe proliferative retinopathy	3 to 4 months
Proliferative retinopathy without high-risk characteristics	2 to 4 months
Proliferative retinopathy with high-risk characteristics	Individualized to patient needs

Assessing Visual Function and Adaptation to Low Vision

1 The individual's functional ability is a reflection of the measurable visual acuity and field as well as the capacity for adaptation to the vision loss.

A Multiple factors influence adaptation to vision loss.

- Individuals with diabetic retinopathy can experience daily fluctuations in vision that may be influenced by postural changes, ambient lighting, and glucose levels. Measurements in the ophthalmologist's office may not reflect the true degree of vision impairment that the patient experiences in other environments.

- Persons who have had time to adapt to vision loss or who have had rehabilitation training may function better in activities of daily living than those who have had less severe vision impairment for a shorter interval. Some totally blind individuals will function more independently than other persons who have an acute milder loss of vision.

B *Visual acuity*, or the sharpness of the central vision, is most often measured through the use of the Snellen chart. Acuity, as defined by the Snellen fraction, is the ratio of the distance at which an individual can read certain letters on the chart compared with the distance required for an individual with normal vision.[24]

- A person with normal vision is said to have 20/20 vision, which means letters intended to be read at 20 ft can be seen at that range.
- An individual with 20/40 vision would need to stand at 20 ft to read letters that a normally sighted person could distinguish at 40 ft.

C The visual field is a measurement of peripheral vision. The normal visual field is 180 degrees. Loss of peripheral vision can cause significant dysfunction despite maintenance of good central visual acuity.[25]

- A decreased visual field may reflect narrowing of the total angle of vision.
- The visual field may also be reduced due to specific blind spots in the central or peripheral vision.

2 Definitions of vision impairment and blindness can vary according to the source.[25,26]

A The American Foundation for the Blind suggests using the term *blind* only for persons who have no usable sight. The term *low vision* is used for persons with some usable vision.

B The term *visually impaired* may apply to persons with all levels of visual disability.

C *Legal blindness* was originally defined by the federal government to denote the level at which individuals are eligible to receive certain benefits. The standard for legal blindness is acuity of less than 20/200 in the better eye with corrective lenses and/or a visual field of less than 20 degrees.

D Standards for mild, moderate, severe, and profound vision impairment are shown in Table 7.4.

3 In addition to assessment of visual acuity and field, the ability to use vision or adaptive alternatives in the practical settings of daily living also needs to be assessed. The following areas need to be addressed.

A Does the patient have adequate vision to perform necessary self-care tasks and use standard instruction materials?[27]

B Does the patient's vision fluctuate? If so, assess all of the following questions for times when the patient's vision is at its worst.

- Can the patient read the lines on a syringe (if using insulin)?
- Can the patient see the display on a blood glucose meter and the spot on which to apply a blood drop?
- Can the patient read standard print or large print, either with or without magnification and appropriate lighting? If not, can the patient use audiotapes or braille?

C If there is inadequate eyesight to perform vision-dependent diabetes self-care skills, is neuromuscular function adequate to acquire tactile skills? Different tactile devices require varying levels of sensory and motor ability.

Table 7.4. Classification of Visual Loss[25]

Classification	Acuity ICD-9[‡]	WHO[*]	Level of Disability
Mild	20/30 to 20/60	<20/25	No special aids necessary
Moderate	20/70 to 20/160	<20/70 or 20/80	Special aids necessary for some tasks (magnification)
Severe	20/200 to 20/400	<20/160	Can read with special aids at reduced speed and endurance
Profound	20/500 to 20/1000	<20/400	Reading and mobility impaired, relies on other senses for some tasks
Near total blindness	—	—	Light perception, relies completely on other senses
Total blindness	—	—	No vision, relies on other senses

[‡]ICD-9 = International Classification of Diseases-9, [*]WHO = World Health Organization

D Does the patient currently need assistance in any of the following areas?
- Shopping and preparing food appropriate to the meal plan
- Walking about the home
- Transportation to medical appointments, social activities, and other activities important to the patient
- Personal hygiene

E Has the patient had any blindness rehabilitation education in daily living skills? Has the patient had any mobility instruction?

F Does the patient have adequate cognitive ability to learn new skills?[27]
- Is the patient so anxious or disoriented by the vision loss that learning a new skill would be extremely difficult? If so, more time may be needed for learning or teaching diabetes skills.
- Has the patient experienced short-term memory loss? If so, does the patient have adequate memory to learn new ways of performing reliable diabetes self-care?

4 Refer patients to appropriate agencies or personnel for a thorough investigation of rehabilitative, psychosocial, and financial needs related to the visual impairment.[27]

A In the US, every state has an agency that provides rehabilitation services to blind people.

B Many cities have private blindness rehabilitation services available from nonprofit agencies.

C The federal Department of Veterans Affairs provides comprehensive blindness rehabilitation services to veterans.

D Call the state information office to find out how to contact the state blindness rehabilitation agent, who will have information about local private agencies and access to veteran's services.

E Information about local services is also available from the American Foundation for the Blind (800-AFBLIND), which maintains a comprehensive referral list. (See additional resources for vision impairment services at the end of this chapter.)

Adaptive Diabetes Education for the Visually Impaired Person

1 Although the goals of diabetes education for persons with visual impairment are the same as for sighted individuals, the content and method of delivery must be adapted to meet their special needs.[27,28]

   A Observe the following rules of courtesy with the patient who is visually impaired.[29]

- Immediately upon entering the room, address the patient by name and introduce yourself using your name and position.
- Use a natural tone and speed in conversation. It is only necessary to speak loudly and slowly when the patient also has a hearing impairment.
- It is acceptable to use words that refer to vision during the conversation: "look," "see," and "watch" are part of everyday conversation. "Blind" and "visually impaired" are not derogatory terms.
- Indicate the end of a conversation and announce if you will be leaving the room. This will prevent any embarrassment to the patient who may continue talking after you have left the room.
- If you need to touch the patient's hands during an equipment demonstration, ask for permission before doing so.

   B Educational materials available in standard print may not be usable by the visually impaired population. There is a lack of accessible diabetes information (audiotaped or braille) available. It may be necessary to record individualized instructions on a cassette.[30]

2 Many adaptive devices are available for the nonvisual measurement of insulin.[31-33]

   A The following options are available for measuring insulin doses.

- For those patients with reliable low vision, using better lighting, contrasting color backgrounds, and/or a magnifier may be all that is necessary. Some magnifiers are made specifically to fit onto the insulin syringe.
- Preset dose gauges are designed to measure the space between the ends of the insulin syringe barrel and the plunger. Commercially prepared gauges are more reliable than those made at home. The patient will require multiple gauges for mixed insulin dosages or for multiple dosages that differ throughout the day.
- A measuring device that holds the insulin vial and syringe can be preset for 1 or 2 doses. The syringe plunger is pulled back to the preset stop, which measures a specific amount of insulin. A sighted individual must preset the doses.
- Variable-dose devices measure insulin for single and mixed doses in 1- and 10-unit increments. Each increment of insulin is measured by clicks that may be felt or heard.
- Several styles of insulin pens are available to measure insulin in 1- or 2-unit increments. Some pens are completely disposable; others use disposable prefilled insulin

cartridges. Both types of devices use a disposable needle. The insulin pens can be operated nonvisually but are not endorsed by the manufacturer for this use.
- At least 1 of the needleless injectors includes tactual and auditory cues for setting the amount of insulin to be delivered.
- Insulin pumps have been used successfully by some patients with visual impairment. Some models come with auditory cues to assist in programming.

B Appropriate equipment is selected based on the treatment plan and motor skills of each patient.
- Only certain insulin-measuring devices are suitable for mixed- and/or variable-dose regimens.
- The size of the insulin dose influences the choice of equipment. Some devices do not measure large doses, and some do not measure 1-unit increments.
- A deficit in fine motor skills or sensory impairment due to neuropathy may prevent the use of certain devices.
- Allow the patient to choose among several suitable devices. Do not assume that one device will be easier to use than another. Provide sufficient time to work with all available equipment, and let patients select the devices which best meet their needs.

C The procedure for using each dose-measuring device differs, although certain principles are universal to their use.
- The insulin vial should first be prepared using the standard method.
- Textured tape, a rubber band, or some other tactile marker on the vial can be used to identify each type of insulin.
- To expel air bubbles from the syringe, pull insulin into the syringe and push it quickly back into the vial at least 3 times before filling the syringe to the desired dose. Tapping the syringe softly at this point will also help to release any trapped air bubbles. When mixing insulin, instruct the patient to follow this procedure with the first insulin; with the second insulin, teach the patient to pull back on the plunger very slowly to prevent air bubbles from entering the syringe. Variable-dose devices may have modified instructions for eliminating air bubbles.
- Observe accurate measurement of insulin using the selected adaptive device at least 3 times on 2 separate occasions before suggesting unsupervised insulin measurement.[34]

D There are several methods to ensure that there is sufficient insulin inside the vial at all times.
- One approach is to determine how many doses that a vial of insulin contains without using the last 50 units of insulin. For example, if the patient takes a total of 40 units each day from a 1000-unit NPH vial, 1 vial of NPH would last 23 days (950 ÷ 40). The patient could set aside 23 syringes and start a new vial when those syringes are used.
- Visually impaired patients can also be taught to shake the insulin vial to determine amount of insulin left. A completely full vial will sound and feel differently than one that is half full or almost empty. Have the visually impaired person practice this method with several vials filled to different levels.

E Review adaptive principles of insulin administration.
- Visually impaired patients can be taught to inject themselves with insulin by using conventional syringes, automatic needle injectors, pen injectors, or needle-free jet injectors.

- When using the conventional syringe without an assistive device, the visually impaired patient is taught to choose the site, pinch the skin, gently place the needle on the skin, and insert the needle into the skin. This method eliminates the usual dart-like motion so that the patient can control where the needle is inserted.
- The injection site is chosen by creating a map of the area to be injected. When creating the map of injection sites, a sighted person can alert the visually impaired person to areas to avoid, such as varicosities and scar tissue.

3 Specialized adaptive equipment is available to assist the patient with visual impairment in blood glucose monitoring.[33-35]

A Evaluate individual needs to assure that the correct adaptive devices are chosen.
- For those with reliable low vision, monitors with large display screens and easy-to-use features may be appropriate. These monitors are made for the general population and are not necessarily marketed for individuals with vision impairment.
- Certain monitors can be adapted with an attachable voice module that verbalizes display messages. This type of monitor is convenient for the patient who is already familiar with the use of the system.
- Certain monitoring systems have been specifically designed for individuals with visual impairment and do not require additional adaptive components. The accuracy of these systems should be verified.[36]

B The techniques for obtaining a blood sample are universal. However, assuring an adequate blood sample and applying that sample to the reagent strip may require adaptive measures.
- The application area of the strip needs to be recognizable by using tactual methods. This task is accomplished by running a finger or fingernail along the edges of the strip to locate distinctive features.
- When checking for an adequate blood drop, patients who bleed easily can touch the puncture site with another finger to feel for wetness. The puncture site also may be touched lightly to the edge of the lip, which is another sensitive area for assessing wetness. Teach patients who find it difficult to obtain an adequate sample methods for increasing blood flow to the finger such as warming the hands before lancing, using a rubberband tourniquet around the finger, and using a lancet cap designed for a deeper penetration. Certain lancet devices allow the user to dial to a deeper penetration setting.
- Some meters have a feature that announces when an adequate blood drop has been applied.
- A few older monitoring systems require blood placement on the strip before it is inserted into the meter. A strip guide can be used to assist in the proper placement of the blood sample.
- Most newer systems allow blood sample placement on the strip after the strip is inserted into the meter. Commercially made blood drop guides can assist with this task. As a less expensive alternative to these devices, raised marks can be added to the monitor on either side of the target area.[28] The tactile marks can be used as a guide for placing the blood drop on the target area.
- One glucose meter uses a curved strip and an electrochemical method for analyzing glucose, allowing placement of blood without an assistive device.

C Tactile labels such as rubberbands or textured tape are useful for identifying various control solutions.

D Because visually impaired patients cannot see when the meter needs to be cleaned, teach them to clean the meter routinely, especially if the blood is applied while the strip is in the meter.

- Certain meters with voice module attachments can "tell" the user that the monitor needs cleaning.
- Meters which use electrochemical analysis do not require cleaning as blood never enters the meter.

4 Proper foot care for the visually impaired patient with diabetes is imperative because of the increased potential for injury and the possible inability to recognize the early signs of infection. It is critical to the patient with visual impairment to learn a nonvisual method of foot inspection.[37-38] The visually impaired patient with diabetes can perform routine foot inspection using the senses of touch, smell, and temperature perception.

A If the sense of touch is reliable, the fingertips can be used to detect changes in the surface of the feet. Teach the patient to notice any breaks in the skin and new callouses, blisters, or objects imbedded in the skin. Teach the patient to inspect the feet on a daily basis, making note of any changes not present the day before.

B The back of the hand can be used to detect changes in temperature.

C When removing shoes and socks, ask the patient to make note of any changes in odor. The sense of smell can be used to detect infections, which can produce a foul odor.

D Patients who are unable to reach their feet, who have neuropathic changes in their hands that affect their sense of touch, or those with an impaired sense of smell will require the assistance of a sighted person to visually inspect their feet.

- Even if the visually impaired patient can reliably perform nonvisual foot assessment, periodic assessment by a sighted person will still be necessary.
- Instruct patients with visual impairment and diabetes not to cut their toenails due to the increased risk of self-inflicted injury. Regular visits to a podiatrist or other foot care specialist are recommended.

5 Exercise recommendations and precautions vary depending upon the degree of vision loss. Visual impairment alone does not prevent a patient from participating in exercise if appropriate adaptations can be made.[39-41]

A Patients with diabetes and proliferative retinopathy will need to take precautions to protect any usable remaining vision.

- There is concern that the increase in systolic blood pressure that occurs during exercise may aggravate underlying eye pathology.
- There is no clear evidence that intensive physical training programs accelerate the progression of diabetic retinopathy. However, certain types of exercises that increase systolic blood pressure with a concomitant increase in intraocular pressure are contraindicated (Table 7.5). See Chapter 2, Exercise, in Diabetes Management Therapies, for more information.

B Exercise routines for the visually impaired patient with diabetes include a warm-up, aerobic activity, and cool down.

- Muscle-stretching exercises such as toe touches can be performed while sitting in a chair and reaching for the extended leg to avoid bending at the waist or lowering head below the heart.

Table 7.5. Exercise Precautions for Patients With Active Diabetic Retinopathy[41]

Avoid activities that involve any of the following:
- Bending over so that the head is positioned lower than the waist
- Valsalva-type maneuvers that raise blood pressure
- Isometric and weight-resistive activities
- Vigorous bouncing (eg, high-impact aerobics)
- Rapid head movements (eg, contact sports or jogging)
- Extreme changes in atmospheric pressure (eg, parachuting or scuba diving)

- For balance, stretching exercises can be done while standing near a wall or heavy chair.
- Walking is a safe and effective aerobic exercise. The patient with visual impairment and diabetes can walk with a sighted guide, on a treadmill, or with a guide rope installed around the yard or along the driveway. Those with adequate training can walk with a white cane or guide dog.
- Many other forms of exercise can be adapted and safely performed by visually impaired people, such as swimming, golfing, tandem bicycle riding, and horseback riding. A newly visually impaired patient who formerly enjoyed a particular form of exercise and wishes to continue it can consult a mobility instructor about possible adaptations.

6 Adaptive devices are available to facilitate food preparation and assist with other diabetes-related activities.

A Adaptive cooking devices include tactile and talking scales, timers, clocks, microwave ovens, and kitchen utensils. Refer the patient to a blindness rehabilitation teacher for individualized instruction in this area.

B To assist with diabetes-related activities, patients can be provided with large-block color comparison charts for ketone testing, talking weight scales, talking sphygmomanometers, talking thermometers, and devices for organizing medications and facilitating the instillation of eye drops.

7 Some diabetes educators specialize in the care and education of visually impaired patients. Educators can refer to the Visually Impaired Specialty Practice Group of the American Association of Diabetes Educators.

Psychosocial Aspects of Diabetes and Vision Loss

1 Visual impairment impacts all aspects of a person's life: family relations, social interactions, finances, employment, and recreation. Visual impairment coupled with diabetes creates added stress and anxiety and can lead to depression. The patient must learn special skills not only to manage everyday activities but also to manage diabetes.[19-20,22,42]

A Diabetes educators are in a key position to direct patients with vision impairment toward the resources they require.[34]

B When vision is lost or severely diminished, routine tasks can cause the greatest frustration. Learning a simple skill, such as pouring a cup of coffee without it overflowing, can provide a patient with the initial self-confidence needed to take on more complicated tasks.

- Rehabilitation is essential for relearning activities of daily living such as safe mobility, household tasks, communication skills, vocational guidance, and education.
- Rehabilitation counseling also can help the patient cope with the impact of visual loss on self-image and relationships.

C Low-vision services have been designed to help a patient use remaining vision more efficiently.

- Many visually impaired patients buy inexpensive magnifiers and are frustrated because the object or print may appear larger but not clearer. Inform patients that more effective options are available, such as audio and tactile devices as well as magnification devices prescribed by a low-vision specialist.
- Low-vision service begins with a comprehensive assessment of the patient's experience, attitude, and adjustment to vision loss. A detailed visual examination focuses on function. The exam is followed by the prescription of low-vision devices (eg, optical lenses) and visual aids (eg, lighting, reading stands, large print). The patient receives training in use of the aids and devices and is reevaluated when necessary.

D The diabetes educator can provide support to the patient with visual impairment and diabetes through active listening; recognizing effective and ineffective coping patterns; and referrals for counseling, rehabilitation, support groups, and education.

- Offer to refer the patient and family members for counseling to adjust to shifting roles and responsibilities within the family.
- The patient may grieve for the many losses associated with vision impairment such as loss of the visual aspects of communication, loss of the pleasure of visual sensory experience, loss of their own sense of personal competence, and loss of body image. If the patient becomes suicidal, or if the grieving is so intense or so prolonged as to interfere with necessary self-care activities, the diabetes educator should make an immediate referral to a mental health professional who is knowledgeable about adjustment to visual impairment.[28,43]
- Often, contact with other people who have adjusted successfully to living with visual impairment can be very helpful to patients with new vision loss. The diabetes educator can refer the patient to peer counseling, support groups, or chapters of the national consumer advocacy organizations if available in the local area.[28]
- The person with visual impairment may need assistance in exploring all financial resources that are available.

Key Educational Considerations

1 Diabetic retinopathy often occurs without any symptoms. Symptoms may not be present until late in the disease process.

A Treatment is most effective when instituted early.

B Patients must understand the importance of having routine dilated eye exams by an eye care specialist.

2 Review the anatomy and function of the eye with the patient. Comparing the eye to a camera is one way to teach this information. The damaged retina can be compared to damaged film in a camera and a cataract to a camera lens with a scratch or crack. This analogy may help the patient understand why stronger refractive lenses may not correct the problem.

3 Instruct patients to immediately report any sudden loss of vision, sudden onset of floaters, the appearance of a shade or curtain coming across the visual field, eye pain, and photophobia to the ophthalmologist.

4 Conventional visual materials will not be useful when teaching patients with total or near-total visual impairment. Most patients may wish to receive audiotapes and a few may be able to use written instructions in braille. Educators have the opportunity to be creative in developing tactile methods of teaching, utilizing plastic food models, raised T-shirt paint, and hands-on demonstrations.

5 Provide and encourage visually impaired patients to explore an adaptive aid with their hands before instruction. The device can then be named and its parts and their location can be described. Use the same name each time when referring to a specific part. Talk with the patient slowly through the entire procedure for using the device.

6 Assist patients to select the syringe-filling device or glucose monitor that will be useful to them if fluctuation or deterioration of vision is anticipated.

Self-Review Questions
1 List 6 risk factors for diabetic retinopathy, in addition to duration of diabetes and glucose control.
2 Define the stages of diabetic retinopathy.
3 Describe the potential consequences of clinically significant macular edema.
4 State the treatment modalities for each stage of diabetic retinopathy.
5 List 7 other ophthalmic complications associated with diabetes.
6 How is visual function determined?
7 Name referral services that can be used by the visually impaired person with diabetes.
8 Describe psychosocial issues that may impact the person with diabetes and visual impairment.
9 List 3 considerations in choosing the appropriate adaptive device for drawing up insulin.
10 List adaptations that will allow persons with diabetes and visual impairment to monitor their glucose level independently.
11 List 2 nonvisual, sensory methods of foot inspection.
12 List 3 adaptive devices to assist in diabetes-related activities of daily living.
13 Describe exercise restrictions that are appropriate for people who have diabetic retinopathy and at least some useful vision.

Learning Assessment: Case Study 1

BW, a 52-year-old woman, went to a neighborhood clinic complaining of blurred vision. She also noticed increased thirst and urination over the past few months. She has not been to a physician in the past few years. Her random blood glucose level was 294 mg/dL (16 mmol/L). The physical examination revealed moderate obesity and a blood pressure of 168/96 mm Hg. The fundus was not sufficiently visible without pupillary dilation. The remainder of the exam was remarkable only for patchy loss of sensation in the lower extremities. Upon referral to an ophthalmologist, she was found to have cotton-wool spots, venous beading, hard exudates, IRMA, and a few small intraretinal (flame) hemorrhages. She was diagnosed as having severe nonproliferative diabetic retinopathy.

Questions for Discussion

1 What should be considered as likely causes of blurred vision in this patient?

2 What is the appropriate treatment for her condition?

3 What adaptations to standard diabetes teaching does this patient need right now?

Discussion

1 This patient has type 2 diabetes of unknown duration. Her blurred vision could be secondary to poor glucose control or serious underlying eye pathology. She needed immediate referral for ophthalmologic evaluation, which in this case revealed severe nonproliferative diabetic retinopathy.

2 In addition to ophthalmoscopy, she will need stereoscopic fundus photography and slitlamp biomicroscopy to evaluate the extent of involvement of the retina and macula. Pan-retinal photocoagulation therapy may be beneficial for severe nonproliferative diabetic retinopathy in this patient with type 2 diabetes, but would be delayed for a type 1 patient until high-risk proliferative retinopathy developed. She will require focal photocoagulation to the macula if clinically significant macular edema is present. Fluorescein angiography would be used to locate specific target lesions and to monitor response to therapy.

3 In addition to immediate attention to her eye problems, she needs to begin an appropriate treatment program for hyperglycemia and hypertension and receive diabetes self-management education. Adjustment to the diagnosis of diabetes and vision impairment needs to be assessed and referrals for counseling or other supportive services offered as needed. This patient is likely to need to learn low-vision methods for blood glucose monitoring, foot inspection, and exercise. If insulin therapy is instituted, she will also need a low vision method for insulin measurement. If the patient has difficulty reading print, provide education materials in large print or audio format.

Learning Assessment: Case Study 2

RI, a 35-year-old man, is referred to you for diabetes self-management education. His home glucose record reveals erratic glycemic control with frequent hypoglycemic episodes. Although RI denies vision impairment, he is unable to accurately draw up his insulin dose when observed. Upon further questioning he reports occasional difficulty reading the newspaper. His physician referred him to an ophthalmologist, but RI has not yet made an appointment.

Questions for Discussion

1 What further assessment of this patient's functional status should be undertaken?

2 What can the diabetes educator do to assist this patient in managing his diabetes?

3 What other services could the diabetes educator recommend to this patient for further assistance?

Discussion

1 This patient appears to have fluctuating vision that is interfering with his diabetes self-care. He is reluctant to acknowledge the visual problem. The patient should be strongly encouraged to undergo a complete ophthalmologic exam to determine if the problem is diabetes related and to ensure that appropriate treatment is initiated. The diabetes educator should assess RI's ability to complete daily activities (driving, working, reading, and personal care tasks) when vision is at its worst.

2 The diabetes educator should further assess RI's diabetes self-care skills, such as glucose monitoring, meal planning, foot care, etc. If he is unable to accurately fill his syringes using a magnifier, the need for an adaptive syringe-filling device is indicated. Although he currently is able to use his glucose meter without difficulty, he can be reassured that there are adaptive devices available to assist with glucose monitoring should there be a change in his vision status.

3 If the assessment shows that RI is having difficulties in other areas due to his visual status, the diabetes educator can make referrals to appropriate rehabilitative or low-vision services. Since he is having difficulty acknowledging his vision problems, the diabetes educator should help explore his fears, provide reassurance, and make referrals for counseling if necessary.

References

1 Javitt JC, Aiello LP. Cost effectiveness of detecting and treating diabetic retinopathy. Ann Intern Med. 1996;124:164-169.

2 Klein R, Klein BEK. Vision disorders in diabetes. In: National Diabetes Data Group, eds. Diabetes in America. 2nd ed. National Institutes of Health; 1995:293-337.

3 Aiello LP, Cavallerano J, Bursell SE. Diabetic eye disease. Endocrinol Metab Clin North Am. 1996;25:271-291.

4 Ferris FL III, Davis MD, Aiello LM. Treatment of diabetic retinopathy [review]. New Engl J Med. 1999; 341:667-678.

5 Aiello LP, Gardner TW, King GL, et al. Diabetic retinopathy (technical review). Diabetes Care. 1998;21:143-156.

6 Williams AS. Visual impairment with diabetes: estimates of lower and upper limits of prevalence in the United States. Diabetes Educ. 1999;25:23-4,27-8.

7 Harris MI. Summary. In: National Diabetes Data Group, eds. Diabetes in America. 2nd ed. National Institutes of Health; 1995:1-13.

8 The Diabetes Control and Complications Trial Research Group. The effect of intensive treatment of diabetes on the development and progression of long-term complications in insulin-dependent diabetes mellitus. N Engl J Med. 1993;329:977-986.

9 UK Prospective Diabetes Study Group. Intensive blood-glucose control with sulphonylureas or insulin compared with conventional treatment and risk of complications in patients with type 2 diabetes (UKPDS 33). Lancet. 1998;352:837-853.

10 UK Prospective Diabetes Study Group. Tight blood pressure control and risk of macrovascular and microvascular complications in type 2 diabetes (UKPDS 38). BMJ. 1998;317:703-713.

11 Chew EY, Klein ML, Ferris FL III, et al. Association of elevated serum lipid levels with retinal hard exudate in diabetic retinopathy: Early Treatment Diabetic Retinopathy Study (ETDRS) report 22. Arch Ophthalmol. 1996;114:1079-1084.

12 Frank KJ, Dieckert JP. Diabetic eye disease: a primary care perspective. South Med J. 1996;89:463-470.

13 Sanders R, Wilson M. Diabetes-related eye disorders. J Natl Med Assoc. 1993; 85:104-108.

14 The Diabetic Retinopathy Study Research Group. Preliminary report on effects of photocoagulation therapy. Am J Ophthalmol. 1976;81:383-396.

15 Early Treatment Diabetic Retinopathy Study Research Group. Photocoagulation for diabetic macular edema. Early Treatment Diabetic Retinopathy Study report 1. Arch Ophthalmol. 1985;103:1796-1806.

16 Ferris F. Early photocoagulation in patients with either type I or type II diabetes. Trans Am Ophthamol Soc. 1996;94:505-537.

17 The Diabetic Retinopathy Vitrectomy Study Research Group. Early vitrectomy for severe vitreous hemorrhage in diabetic retinopathy: two-year results of a randomized trial: Diabetic Retinopathy Vitrectomy Study report 2. Arch Ophthalmol. 1985;103:1644-1652.

18 Bernbaum M, Albert SG. Referring patients with diabetes and vision loss for rehabilitation—who is responsible? Diabetes Care. 1996;19:175-177.

19 Bernbaum M, Albert SG, Duckro PN. Psychosocial profiles in patients with visual impairment due to diabetic retinopathy. Diabetes Care. 1988;11:551-557.

20 Jacobson AM. Current concepts: the psychological care of patients with insulin-dependent diabetes mellitus. N Engl J Med. 1996;334:1249-1253.

21 Wulsin LR, Jacobson AM, Rand LI. Psychosocial adjustment to advanced proliferative diabetic retinopathy. Diabetes Care. 1993;16:1061-1066.

22 Cox DJ, Kiernan BD, Schroeder DB, Cowley M. Psychosocial sequelae of visual loss in diabetes. Diabetes Educ. 1998; 24:481-484.

23 American Academy of Ophthalmology Quality of Care Committee Retina Panel. Preferred Practice Pattern for Diabetic Retinopathy. San Francisco: American Academy of Ophthalmology; 1993.

24 Collins JF. Ophthalmic Desk Reference. New York: Raven Press; 1991:615.

25 Simons K. Visual acuity and the functional definition of blindness. In: Tasman W, Jaeger EA, eds. Duane's Clinical Ophthalmology. Philadelphia: Lippincott; 1991:1-21.

26 American Foundation for the Blind. Low Vision Questions and Answers: Definitions, Devices, Services. New York: American Foundation for the Blind; 1987.

27 William AS, Teaching nonvisual diabetes self-care: choosing appropriate tools and techniques for visually impaired individuals. Diabetes Spectrum. 1997;10:128-134.

28 Bernbaum M, Wittry S, Stich T, Brusca S, Albert S. Effectiveness of a diabetes education program adapted for people with vision impairment. Diabetes Care. 2000:23:1430-1432.

29 American Foundation for the Blind. Sensitivity to Blindness and Visual Impairment. New York: American Foundation for the Blind; 1991.

30 Williams AS. Accessible diabetes education materials in low-vision format. Diabetes Educ. 1999;25:695-704.

31 American Diabetes Association Resource Guide 2000: Aids for People Who Are Visually or Physically Impaired. Diabetes Forecast (Suppl) 2000:38-41.

32 Petzinger RA. Adaptive medication measurement and administration. In: Cleary M, ed. Diabetes and Visual Impairment: An Educators Resource Guide. Chicago: American Association of Diabetes Educators Education and Research Foundation, 1994:121-142.

33 Williams AS. Recommendations for desirable features of adaptive diabetes self-care equipment for visually impaired persons. Diabetes Care. 1994;17:451-452.

34 ADEVIP Task Force. Guidelines for the practice of adaptive diabetes education for visually impaired persons (ADEVIP). Diabetes Educ. 1994;20:111-112,115-116, 118.

35 Petzinger RA. Adaptive self-monitoring strategies. In: Cleary M, ed. Diabetes and Visual Impairment: An Educators Resource Guide. Chicago: American Association of Diabetes Educators Education and Research Foundation; 1994:143-157.

36 Bernbaum SM, Albert SG, Miller D, Hoffman JW, Mooradian AD. Reliability of the Diascan Partner glucose monitor for visually impaired people. Diabetes Spectrum. 1995;8:322-324.

37 Plummer E, Albert SG. Foot care assessment in patients with diabetes: a screening algorithm for patient education and referral. Diabetes Educ. 1995; 21:47-51.

38 Williams A. Foot care for the visually impaired. Diabetes Self Manage. 1992; 9(6):41-43.

39 Albert SG, Bernbaum M. Exercise for patients with diabetic retinopathy. Diabetes Care. 1995;18:130-132.

40 Bernbaum M. Adaptive exercise recommendations. In: Cleary M, ed. Diabetes and Visual Impairment: An Educators Resource Guide. Chicago: American Association of Diabetes Educators Education and Research Foundation; 1994:111-119.

41 Graham C, Lasko-McCarthey P. Exercise options for persons with diabetic complications. Diabetes Educ. 1990;16:212-220.

42Bernbaum M, Albert SG, Duckro PN, Merkel W. Personal and family stress in individuals with diabetes and vision loss. J Clin Psychol. 1993;49:670-677.

43Carroll TJ, Blindness: What It Is, What It Does, And How to Live With It. Boston: Little, Brown & Co; 1961.

Suggested Readings

American Diabetes Association. Diabetic retinopathy (position statement). Diabetes Care. 2001;24(Suppl 1):S73-S76.

Bernbaum M, Albert SG, Brusca SR, et al. A model clinical program for patients with diabetes and vision impairment. Diabetes Educ. 1989;15:325-330.

Cleary M, ed. Diabetes and Visual Impairment: An Educators Resource Guide. Chicago: American Association of Diabetes Educators Education and Research Foundation; 1994:121-142.

Greenblatt S, ed. Meeting the Needs of People With Vision Loss. Lexington, Ma: Resources for Rehabilitation; 1991.

IDF Consultative Section on Diabetes Education. Position Statement on Diabetes Education for People Who Are Blind or Visually Impaired. International Consensus Position Statements for Diabetes Education; 2000:62-72.

Other Resources

Consumer and service organizations
American Council of the Blind
1155 Fifteenth Street, NW, Suite 1004
Washington, DC 20005
202-467-5081
800-424-8666
www.acb.org

American Foundation for the Blind
11 Penn Plaza, Suite 300
New York, NY 10001
212-504-7600
800-232-5463
www.afb.org

LIONS Club International
300 West Twenty-Second Street
Oakbrook, IL 60523
630-571-5466
www.lions.org

National Eye Institute
Information Officer
Building 31, Room 6A32
Bethesda, MD 20205
301-496-5248
www.nei.nih.gov

National Federation of the Blind*
1800 Johnson Street
Baltimore, MD 21230
410-659-9314
www.nfb.org

Prevent Blindness America
500 East Remington Road
Schaumburg, IL 60173
847-843-2020
800-331-2020
www.preventblindness.org

Sources for audiotaped and braille reading material
American Printing House for the Blind
1839 Frankfort Avenue
Louisville, KY 40206
502-895-2405
800-223-1839
www.aph.org

National Library Service for the Blind
and Physically Handicapped
Library of Congress
1291 Taylor Street, NW
Washington, DC 20542
202-287-510
800-424-8567
www.lcweb.loc.gov/nls

Recording for the Blind and Dyslexic
20 Roszel Road
Princeton, NJ 08540
800-221-4792
www.rfbd.org

Correspondence Courses
(including courses on diabetes and
adjustment to vision loss)
Hadley School for the Blind
700 Elm Street
Winnetka, IL 60093
847-446-8111
800-323-4238
www.hadley/school.org

*A Braille Exchange List (ADA Diet-1995) and a comprehensive listing of diabetes products for people with vision impairment are available from the National Federation of the Blind. (See above listing for contact information.)

Learning Assessment: Post-Test Questions

Eye Disease and Adaptive Diabetes Education for Visually Impaired Persons

7

1 Neovascularization that covers 25% or more of the optic disk is characteristic of:
  A Severe nonproliferative retinopathy
  B Clinically significant macular edema
  C Less than high-risk proliferative retinopathy
  D High-risk proliferative diabetic retinopathy

2 For a person with visual impairment to be categorized as legally blind, he or she would have to have:
  A A visual acuity that is <20/80 in the better eye with corrective lenses and/or a visual field of <40 degrees
  B A visual acuity that is <20/160 in the better eye with corrective lenses and/or a visual field of <30 degrees
  C A visual acuity that is <20/200 in the better eye with corrective lenses and/or a visual field < 20 degrees
  D The level of disability in which the individual has no light perception

3 Which type of activity should not be recommended to a patient with active diabetic retinopathy?
  A Jogging
  B Warm ups
  C Walking
  D Modified stretching

4 MB, a newly diagnosed patient with type 2 diabetes, needs referral for a routine ophthalmologic screening and follow-up:
  A Annually, beginning at the time diabetes is diagnosed
  B Semiannually, beginning 2 years after the time that diabetes was diagnosed
  C Every 4 to 6 months, beginning 5 years after the time that diabetes was diagnosed
  D Wait until visual changes occur and then begin to schedule semi-annually

5 Ocular conditions with increased incidence in people with diabetes include all of the following except:
  A Cataracts
  B Retinitis pigmentosa
  C Glaucoma
  D Ocular palsies

6 Treatment of mild-to-moderate retinopathy includes all of the following except:
  A Normalizing blood glucose levels
  B Monitoring blood pressure
  C Smoking cessation
  D In-office laser treatments

7 TS, a 52-year-old blind woman with diabetes, is being taught to calculate and plan for the number of days a vial of insulin will last. TC uses a total of 35 units of NPH insulin once a day. How many syringes should she use before starting a new vial and setting aside a new batch of syringes?
  A 25
  B 27
  C 29
  D 31

8 An adaptive insulin administration aid for the visually impaired:
  A Should be selected by the diabetes educator
  B Is selected based only on the size of the insulin dose
  C Is selected based on the patient's tactile ability and preference
  D Is selected based on the patient's best corrected vision

9 Which of the following is not a condition known to increase the risk for diabetic retinopathy?
  A Uncontrolled blood pressure
  B Pregnancy
  C Renal failure
  D Age less than 10

10 All of the following are important adaptive features to assist the visually impaired in glucose monitoring except:
  A Attachable voice modules
  B A tactile feature indicating the reactive area of the strip
  C Oversized glucose meters that are not easily misplaced
  D Glucose meters that give an audible signal when an appropriate blood sample is applied

See next page for answer key.

Post-Test Answer Key

Eye Disease and Adaptive Diabetes Education for Visually Impaired Persons

7

1   D

2   C

3   A

4   A

5   B

6   D

7   B

8   C

9   D

10 C

A Core Curriculum for Diabetes Education
Diabetes and Complications

Nephropathy 8

Beth Ann Coonrod, PhD, MPH, RN, CDE
Heritage Valley Health System
Beaver and Sewickley, Pennsylvania

Kristina L. Ernst, BSN, RN, CDE
Atlanta, Georgia

Introduction

1 The spectrum of renal changes that occur in individuals with diabetes and that can not be ascribed to other causes is known as *diabetic nephropathy*. At the severe end of this spectrum is overt (or clinically apparent) diabetic nephropathy, which is characterized by persistent proteinuria (>0.5 g/24 h), hypertension, and a progressive decline in renal function that often leads to end-stage renal disease (ESRD) and/or premature mortality from cardiovascular disease. Toward the milder end of the spectrum is *microalbuminuria,* an increase in the urinary albumin excretion (AER) >20 µg/min but ≤200 µg/min (which is approximated by the range of 30 to 300 mg/24 h).

2 Diabetes has become the most common single cause of ESRD in the US and Europe.[1,2] In the US, diabetic nephropathy accounts for about one third of all cases of ESRD. The cost for treatment of patients with diabetes and ESRD is in excess of $2 billion annually.

3 About 20% to 30% of persons with type 1 or type 2 diabetes develop evidence of nephropathy. In individuals with type 1 diabetes, it is the leading cause of death[3-6] and a major risk factor for cardiovascular disease.[6-9] Individuals with type 1 diabetes have an incidence of ESRD greater than 11 to 15 times the incidence found in individuals with type 2 diabetes.[10,11] However, given the greater prevalence of type 2 diabetes, over half of those patients with diabetes currently starting on dialysis have type 2 diabetes.[1]

  A Racial/ethnic differences also exist; incidence rates for African Americans, Hispanics (especially Mexican Americans), and Native Americans are 3 to 6 times higher than rates among non-Hispanic Caucasians with type 2 diabetes.[1]

  B The growth in the number of ESRD patients has been particularly dramatic in the elderly. Individuals over age 60 years represent 55% of all incident cases.

4 Studies have demonstrated that the onset and course of diabetic nephropathy can be ameliorated by several interventions, including attaining and maintaining glycemic and blood pressure control, using antihypertensive agents, and decreasing dietary protein intake.[1] These interventions have their greatest impact if instituted very early in the course of this complication, highlighting the importance of detecting microalbuminuria before diabetic nephropathy is clinically evident.

5 For patients who experience renal failure, several possible treatment modalities exist. Individual needs must be considered when deciding which of the following treatment options to pursue.

  A No therapy (resulting in death)

  B Hemodialysis

  C Peritoneal dialysis

  D Kidney transplant

  E Simultaneous kidney-pancreas transplant

6 Caring for patients with diabetic nephropathy is challenging and requires expertise of a variety of disciplines (eg, medicine, mental health, nursing, nutrition, pharmacy, social services), which must integrate renal and diabetes care. Surgery and rehabilitation services may be necessary for patients who progress to renal failure.

Objectives

Upon completion of this chapter, the learner will be able to:

1 Discuss the epidemiology of diabetic nephropathy and end-stage renal disease.

2 Describe the basic functions of the kidney.

3 Describe the major stages in the natural progression of diabetic nephropathy.

4 List diagnostic tests used to assess and monitor renal function.

5 Review treatment modalities for diabetic nephropathy.

6 List treatment options for renal replacement therapy.

7 Identify prevention strategies and when they should be implemented.

Key Definitions

1 *Albumin.* The major plasma protein. Albumin is generally too large to be filtered out of the blood as it passes through the glomeruli; thus, it is normally found in only minute amounts in the urine. Increased amounts of albumin in the urine indicate glomerular damage.

2 *Albumin excretion rate (AER).* The amount of albumin that is excreted in the urine over a given period. AER is commonly expressed in μg/min or mg/24 h. An increase in the AER can indicate an abnormality at the glomerular filter that is allowing albumin to enter the filtrate in greater amounts.

3 *Bowman capsule.* A cuplike structure that surrounds the glomerulus.

4 *Blood urea nitrogen (BUN).* The blood level of urea. Urea is the end product of protein metabolism and is formed in the liver. After synthesis, urea travels through the blood and is excreted in the urine. The normal plasma value of urea is 8 to 20 mg/dL (2.9 to 7.1 mmol/L), varying with the quantity and quality of protein intake, state of hydration, and kidney function. The blood level rises as kidney function deteriorates.

5 *Creatinine (Cr).* A nitrogen compound formed mainly from the metabolism of muscle. An individual's daily production rate of creatinine is relatively constant. The normal plasma value is 0.5 to 1.4 mg/dL (44 to 124 μmol/L), varying with body size and gender; males have higher levels than females. Serum creatinine rises as kidney function deteriorates, but not indefinitely (ie, it will eventually stabilize despite continued deterioration of renal function).

6 *Creatinine clearance (CrCl).* CrCl measures the rate at which creatinine is removed from the blood by the kidney and is used as an estimate of the glomerular filtration rate (GFR) and an approximate measure of kidney function. CrCl compares the amount of creatinine in a serum or plasma sample with the amount found in a timed urine specimen, which approximates how much creatinine the kidneys filter out of the blood each minute. Most people clear about 100 to 125 mg/min. A fall in CrCl is a sign of declining renal function. However, as the true GFR decreases in renal disease, the estimation of GFR by CrCl becomes uncertain.

7 *End-stage renal disease (ESRD).* The term used to describe advanced kidney failure. Renal replacement therapy (eg, dialysis or transplantation) must be implemented for life to continue.

8 *Microalbuminuria.* An increase in the urinary AER above normal but below the level of overt proteinuria. More specifically, microalbuminuria is defined as an AER >20 µg/min but ≤200 µg/min (which is approximated by 30 to 300 mg/24 h).[12] There is a large intraindividual day-to-day variation in AER in individuals with diabetes.[13-17] Therefore, the absence or presence of microalbuminuria should be determined based on more than one urine collection.

9 *Glomerulus.* The filtering component of the nephron. It is a tuft of capillaries in which filtration of blood takes place. A kidney biopsy will show structural changes in the glomeruli of a patient with diabetic nephropathy.

10 *Glomerular basement membrane.* A selectively permeable structure located between the glomerular capillaries and the Bowman capsule that serves as a dialyzing membrane to regulate the passage of water and solutes.

11 *Glomerular filtration.* A process that initiates the production of urine with the formation of an ultrafiltrate as blood passes through the glomerular capillaries. Glomerular filtration is governed by a number of factors, including the anatomy of the glomerulus and its Bowman capsule (eg, the size of the pores and the electrical charges within the glomerular filter and the relative diameters of the afferent and efferent arterioles).

12 *Glomerular filtration rate (GFR).* The rate at which the kidney produces glomerular filtrate. GFR represents the amount of fluid that passes from the blood into the capsular space over a given period of time. Normal GFR is approximately 100 to 125 mL/min. This rate is determined using a precise technique that measures the renal clearance of a marker substance; GFR values are used primarily in research. GFR decreases with aging, the presence of kidney or vascular diseases, sodium and water depletion, hemorrhage, and vigorous exercise. The rate increases with dietary protein intake, hyperglycemia, and pregnancy. Repeated measurements of GFR over time provide more useful information than a single value.

13 *Mesangium.* The central core tissue in the glomerulus, bounded by the capillary endothelium and the glomerular basement membrane. The mesangium may play a role in regulating glomerular blood flow.

14 *Nephrons.* The functional units of the kidneys that serve to clear the blood of waste materials and form urine. Each kidney contains about 1 million nephrons. Each nephron consists of a glomerulus leading to a long tubule in which the filtrate is concentrated and modified before it is eliminated as urine.

15 *Nephrotic syndrome.* A state characterized by urinary protein excretion >3.5 g/24 h (which roughly corresponds to an AER >2400 µg/min). Typically, the rate of protein excretion can increase from 4 to 30 g/24 h, resulting in low blood protein levels and massive fluid retention. Hypertension, weight gain, peripheral edema, hyper-lipidemia, hyperfibrinogenemia, hypercoagulability, increased blood viscosity, congestive heart failure, and pulmonary edema are common clinical manifestations of the nephrotic syndrome. Although many people with diabetes manifest nephrotic range proteinuria, true nephrotic syndrome occurs in only 10% to 20% of patients.

16 *Proteinuria.* The presence of protein in the urine. While the degree of proteinuria is often assessed by concentration, it is more precisely measured when quantified as the amount of protein excreted over a given period of time. The normal amount of protein excreted is approximately 0.1 g/24 h. Excess amounts of protein are pathologic, indicating either systemic disease or kidney disease. Overt proteinuria is indicated by the excretion of albumin at a rate >200 µg/min (300 mg/24 h) or by the excretion of >0.5 g of total protein in 24 h.

17 *Uremia.* A syndrome characteristic of ESRD that develops as renal function declines, causing an accumulation of urea, creatinine, and other metabolic waste products in the blood. This extra amount of urea results in anemia, osteodystrophy, neuropathy, and acidosis. Nausea, hypertension, susceptibility to infection, and generalized organ dysfunction frequently accompany this syndrome.

18 *Urinary albumin/creatinine ratio (A/C ratio).* The ratio of the urinary albumin concentration to the urinary creatinine concentration. Use of the A/C ratio can help to reduce inaccuracies that can occur in assessing albumin excretion based on concentration alone — inaccuracies (particularly false negative results) that especially can occur in individuals with diabetes whose urinary volume, and possibly concentration, can vary depending on the degree of glucosuria and polyuria. A/C ratios, however, have been shown to have little or no less intraindividual day-to-day variation than AERs.[14,15,17] The A/C ratio of a midmorning single-void urine sample collected after initial morning voiding has been shown to be both highly correlated with and highly predictive of an individual's AER measured from a 24-h urine collection.[18] This test is often found to be the easiest to carry out in an office setting.

Renal Physiology

1 Normally, people have two kidneys located posterior to the abdominal cavity. Each kidney is the size and shape of an Idaho potato, weighs approximately 5 oz (150 g), and contains about 1 million nephrons.

2 Urine formation begins in the glomerulus. Blood from the systemic circulation enters each glomerulus through its afferent arteriole and exits through its efferent arteriole. The kidneys help to maintain the internal environment of the body by regulating the quality of plasma.

3 Blood flow to the kidneys is approximately 1300 mL/min and accounts for 25% of the cardiac output.

4 The kidney, which is an excretory organ, performs several important metabolic and endocrine functions:[19]

A Removal of water, urea, creatinine, and other metabolic wastes and toxins from the body (ie, formation of urine)

B Maintenance of blood volume

C Preservation of acid-base and electrolyte (sodium, potassium) balance

D Regulation of blood pressure

E Synthesis of erythropoietin, a hormone that stimulates and regulates the production of red blood cells

F Formation of 1,25 dehydroxy vitamin D

Incidence and Prevalence of Diabetic Nephropathy

1 US Renal Data Systems (USRDS) collects information about ESRD in the US.[19]

   A Diabetes is the most common cause of ESRD in the US.

   B There are currently over 80 500 prevalent cases of ESRD in the US caused by diabetes, accounting for 30% to 40% of all new cases of ESRD.[19]

   C Over 15 000 new patients are enrolled in the ESRD program annually.

   D The incidence rate of ESRD among patients with diabetes has been increasing at a striking rate.

2 Diabetic nephropathy develops in 40% to 50% of persons with type 1 diabetes who have had diabetes for greater than 20 years.[20] Individuals who do not develop microalbuminuria or other clinical signs of nephropathy after 25 to 30 years of diabetes are less likely to develop nephropathy. Figure 8.1 depicts the natural history of nephropathy in persons with type 1 diabetes. Microalbuminuria is detected approximately 5 to 8 years before the onset of overt proteinuria.[21]

3 Clinically significant renal disease is less common in type 2 diabetes, occurring in 5% to 10%. However, because of the much greater prevalence of type 2 diabetes, patients with type 2 diabetes constitute over half of those patients with diabetes starting on dialysis.[1]

   A African Americans with diabetes are 4 to 5 times more likely to develop ESRD than Caucasians with diabetes.[19,22]

   B Hispanics and Native Americans have an incidence of diabetic ESRD that is 6.3 times higher than Caucasians with diabetes.[22]

4 The natural history of nephropathy in type 2 diabetes is less well defined than in type 1 diabetes. Uncertain duration of diabetes and coexisting conditions, including hypertension, make it more difficult to isolate the role of diabetes in ESRD in type 2 diabetes.

   A In some individuals, microalbuminuria or proteinuria is present at the time of diagnosis of type 2 diabetes, perhaps reflecting a long period of unrecognized hyperglycemia.

   B The morphological changes in type 2 diabetic nephropathy are also similar to those of type 1 and include renal hypertrophy, glomerular basement membrane thickening, mesangial expansion, and nodular intercapillary glomerulosclerosis (*Kimmelstiel-Wilson lesion*).

Figure 8.1. Natural History of Nephropathy in Type 1 Diabetes

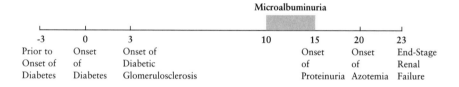

-3	0	3	Time, yr	15	20	23
120	150	150	GFR, mL/min	120	60	<10
1.0	0.8	0.8	Serum Creatinine, mg/dL	1.0	>2.0	>10
15	10	10	Serum Urea Nitrogen, mg/dL	15	>30	<100

Microalbuminuria

-3	0	3	10	15	20	23
Prior to Onset of Diabetes	Onset of Diabetes	Onset of Diabetic Glomerulosclerosis		Onset of Proteinuria	Onset of Azotemia	End-Stage Renal Failure

Source: Reprinted with permission from DeFronzo.[21]

Stages in the Development of Renal Changes

1 Five distinct stages of renal changes in the course of diabetic nephropathy in type 1 diabetes have been proposed.[23,24] (Table 8.1) It should be noted, however, that several studies have reported findings that do not fit this model and suggest a multifactorial etiology of diabetic nephropathy and great variability among individuals in the rate of development and progression of this complication. In addition, differences are likely to exist in the development and progression of this complication between individuals with type 1 diabetes and those with type 2 diabetes.

Table 8.1. Stages of Renal Disease in Patients With Type 1 Diabetes

Stage	Characteristics	Onset	% Progressing to Next Stage (without treatment)
1	*Functional changes* • Early hypertrophy and hyperfiltration	Onset of diabetes	100%
2	*Structural changes* • Renal lesions	2 to 3 years	35% to 40%
3	*Incipient nephropathy*	7 to 15 years	80% to 100%
4	*Overt nephropathy* • Proteinuria	10 to 30 years	50% to 75%
5	*End-stage renal disease*	20 to 40 years	75% to 100%

Source: Adapted from Mogensen[23] and Selby.[24]

A Stage 1 is characterized by hyperfiltration and renal hypertrophy.
  - These changes frequently are seen at the time of diagnosis of diabetes.
  - Near-normal glycemic control at this stage has been shown to restore alterations in kidney function and size.

B Stage 2 involves structural changes, including glomerular basement membrane thickening and mesangial expansion.
  - Renal hyperfunction and hypertrophy are detectable on biopsy and progress silently over several years.[23]
  - These structural changes appear to initiate the decline in renal function. GFR is elevated and may be related to suboptimal glycemic control.

C Stage 3, incipient diabetic nephropathy, develops after 7 to 15 years of diabetes duration when microalbuminuria first appears.
  - Functional and structural renal alterations lead to abnormal filtration of microscopic amounts of protein into the urine. Just when in the development of diabetic nephropathy the decline in GFR begins is unclear. Mogensen and Christensen reported that the GFR and AER increase concomitantly until the GFR exceeds 150 mL/min and the AER reaches 30 µg/min, after which the GFR declines while the AER continues to increase.[25]
  - Blood pressure during this stage may be normal or slightly elevated; patients are generally asymptomatic.
  - The presence of microalbuminuria in type 1 diabetes appears to be a strong predictor of clinical or overt diabetic nephropathy.[25-28]

D Stage 4 is overt (clinical) diabetic nephropathy.
  - Abnormal filtration of protein increases progressively and becomes persistent in this stage.
  - Nephrotic syndrome and hypertension are usually present. Suboptimal blood pressure and glucose control are positively correlated with the rate of GFR decline.

E Stage 5, end-stage renal disease, develops in 75% to 100% of patients with overt nephropathy within 20 years.[1]
  - GFR is less than 15 mL/min and uremia is present.
  - Usually, patients with a serum creatinine level >5 mg/dL (>442 µmol/L) are unable to resume their normal activities because of signs and symptoms of uremia (Table 8.2).
  - Patients with diabetes are clinically sicker at equivalent levels of kidney dysfunction than patients without diabetes.

Other Considerations in the Progression of Renal Disease

1 One fourth to one third of injected insulin is catabolized by the kidney. As kidney function declines, exogenous insulin acts longer and in an unpredictable manner, characterized by recurrent or severe hypoglycemia in some patients. The use of multiple daily insulin injections and hypoglycemia awareness training may reduce the frequency and severity of hypoglycemic episodes.

2 Management and rehabilitation of these patients are further complicated by the fact that more than 95% of patients with diabetic nephropathy have some degree of retinopathy, with 50% being blind or having lost significant vision (renal-retinal syndrome).

Table 8.2. Signs and Symptoms of Uremia

- Anorexia
- Nausea
- Vomiting
- Anemia
- Acidosis

- Pruritus
- Dyspnea
- Lethargy
- Hypertension
- Fluctuating blood glucose levels

3 The prognostic significance of microalbuminuria and proteinuria in patients with type 2 diabetes indicates increased cardiovascular mortality.[29,30]

4 Seventy percent to 80% of patients with diabetes do not develop ESRD and may live without significant renal complications throughout their lives.[1,19]

Pathogenesis of Diabetic Nephropathy

1 Hyperglycemia plays a role in the pathogenesis of diabetic nephropathy.
   A Alteration in tubuloglomerular feedback occurs, resulting in renal vasodilation, increased renal blood flow, and hyperfiltration.
   B Abnormalities in polyol (eg, sorbitol) metabolism occur.
   - Because the kidney does not require insulin for glucose uptake, excess glucose in renal tissue is metabolized by aldose reductase through the polyol pathway to sorbitol. This action initiates a chain of biochemical alterations that lead to depletion of tissue myoinositol concentrations in the glomerulus.
   C Accelerated formation of nonenzymatic advanced glycosylation end products (AGEs) in tissues is directly correlated with hyperglycemia.
   - An increase in circulating AGE peptides parallels the severity of renal dysfunction in diabetic nephropathy.
   - Glycosylation of proteins in the capillary basement membrane may stimulate mesangial growth leading to mesangial expansion.
   - Glycation of albumin can also contribute to its loss across the glomerular basement membrane.

2 Other hormonal imbalances, aside from insufficient insulin, have been implicated in the pathogenesis of diabetic nephropathy.
   A Growth hormone and glucagon, which are both elevated in poorly controlled diabetes, have been shown to produce glomerular hyperfiltration.
   B Increased levels of atrial natriuretic factor (ANF) may also contribute to glomerular hyperfiltration, perhaps as a result of chronic plasma volume expansion.
   C Changes in circulating levels of angiotensin II, catecholamines, and prostaglandins, or altered responsiveness to these vasoactive hormones, may also result in hyperfiltration. It is theorized that angiotensin II may promote cellular and glomerular hypertrophy as well as mesangial expansion.[31]

3 Renal hemodynamic changes play a role in the pathogenesis of diabetic nephropathy. Defects in glomerular cellular metabolism lead to hemodynamic changes in the kidney.[32]

A Glomerular hypertension contributes to increased pressure and flow across the glomerular membrane, resulting in hyperfiltration.

B Glomerular hypertension and the associated renal vasodilation and hyperfiltration increase glomerular protein filtration, leading to proteinuria and mesangial deposition of circulating proteins.

C Mesangial expansion and glomerulosclerosis result in destruction of nephrons. Unaffected nephrons must then work harder.

D In response to the destruction of nephrons, a positive feedback stimulus for compensatory hyperfiltration is initiated, with further increasing single-nephron GFR and progressive renal injury.

E Self-destruction of the surviving glomeruli occurs. Glomerular hypertension mediates the progressive destruction of nephrons.[33]

Risk Factors for Diabetic Nephropathy

1 Multiple factors have been identified that place individuals at increased risk of diabetic nephropathy, including hypertension, poor glycemic control, genetic predisposition, and smoking. A high intake of dietary protein has also been proposed as a risk factor. However, dietary intake of protein is reported to be similar in patients with or without nephropathy.[34] No single risk factor is consistently associated with all cases; a combination of risk factors are likely to be responsible for increasing the risk for diabetic nephropathy.

A Hypertension is twice as prevalent among individuals with type 1 and type 2 diabetes than in the nondiabetic population.

- Diabetic nephropathy increases the risk of hypertension, and hypertension exacerbates the progression of diabetic nephropathy.[35]
- Clinical hypertension is uncommon at the time of diagnosis of type 1 diabetes, whereas blood pressure is frequently elevated at the time of diagnosis in type 2 diabetes.
- Adequate systemic blood pressure control[36] and use of angiotensin-converting enzyme (ACE) inhibitors have been shown to independently reduce the rate of progression of early diabetic renal disease in randomized, controlled trials of persons with type 2 diabetes.[37,38]

B Hyperglycemia is one of the most important risk factors for persistent proteinuria. The rate of progression of diabetic nephropathy in type 1 diabetes can be significantly reduced by optimizing glycemic control, as evidenced in the Diabetes Control and Complications Trial (DCCT)[39] and the Stockholm Diabetes Intervention Study.[40] A pioneer study in persons with type 2 diabetes reported similar outcomes.[41] This was confirmed by the United Kingdom Prospective Diabetes Study, which documented the association between hyperglycemia and microvascular complications in persons with type 2 diabetes.[42]

C In studies in people with type 1 and type 2 diabetes, no evidence supports the claim that protein intake <20% of total energy intake contributes to the development of renal disease.[43-47]

- Protein intake is reported to be similar in persons who do or do not develop diabetic nephropathy with no correlation between protein intake and clinical proteinuria.
- A cross-sectional study of more than 2,500 persons with type 1 diabetes reported that protein consumption of <20% of total energy resulted in average AERs below 20 µg/min.[48] However, in those in whom protein intake was >20% of energy, average AERs increased and were in the microalbuminuric range. Therefore, it may be prudent to limit protein intake to <20% of energy.

D Studies that have examined smoking and proteinuria in individuals with diabetes have rather consistently shown a relationship to exist between these 2 variables.[49-52]

E There are several nonmodifiable risk factors for diabetic nephropathy:
- Increased duration of diabetes is the most important risk factor for the development of nephropathy.[53-56]
- Younger age at diagnosis has been shown to be related to an increased incidence of nephropathy.[6,9,54] However, not all studies agree.[57]
- Some[5,6,54,58] but not all[57] studies have shown a preponderance of nephropathy among men compared to women. Orchard et al[53] reported an excess of diabetic nephropathy in men but indicated that the male excess did not occur until after 25 years of diabetes.
- A positive family history of hypertension has been associated with a greater prevalence of nephropathy.[59,60] However, as higher blood pressure has been found among individuals with a positive family history of hypertension,[61-64] it may be that this relationship actually is reflecting an association between predisposition to hypertension and diabetic nephropathy.
- A positive family history of diabetic nephropathy has been shown to be a risk factor for diabetic nephropathy, but it is unclear whether this clustering of nephropathy within families is due to genetic or environmental influences.[65,66]

Diagnosis and Renal Function Tests

1 Individuals are asymptomatic throughout the early stages of diabetic nephropathy.

2 Diagnostic tests focus on early detection of microalbuminuria.

A Annual screening for microalbuminuria in type 1 diabetes should begin with puberty and after a 5-year disease duration. Among people with type 2 diabetes, screening for microalbuminuria should begin at the time of diagnosis (Figure 8.2).[1] Screening for microalbuminuria can be performed by 3 methods:
- Measurement of the albumin-to-creatinine ratio in a random spot urine collection
- 24-hour urine collection with creatinine, allowing simultaneous measurement of creatinine clearance
- Timed (eg, 4-hour or overnight) collection

B Creatinine clearance (CrCl) is the most widely used direct method of estimating GFR. This value is measured based on results of a carefully timed urine collection, usually over 24 hours.

C Serum creatinine (SCr) is an indirect measurement of GFR. Subtle changes in serum creatinine (eg, 0.8 to 1.3 mg/dL) may in fact indicate major functional loss and should command attention.

Figure 8.2. Screening for Microalbuminuria

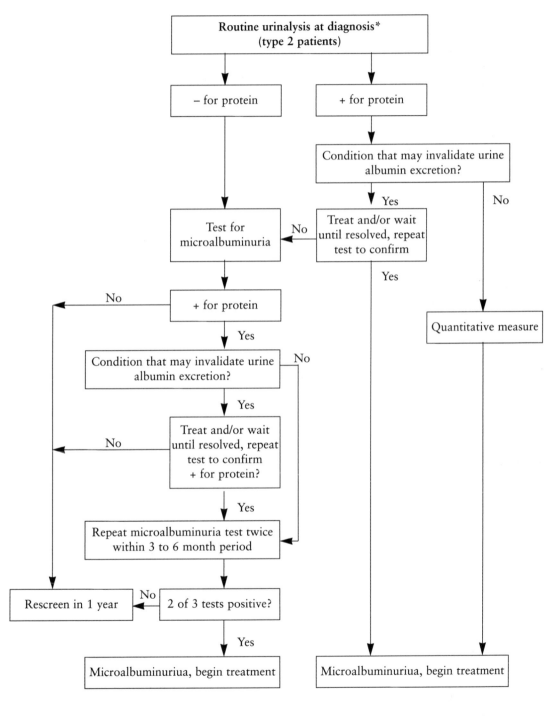

*In type 1 diabetes, screening for albuminuria should begin with puberty and after 5 years' disease duration.

Source: Reprinted with permission from the American Diabetes Association.[1]

- It is well accepted that changes in SCr between 1.4 mg/dL and 6.0 to 7.0 mg/dL parallel changes in GFR as measured by insulin clearance.[67]

D Blood urea nitrogen (BUN) is an indirect measurement of GFR.

- BUN is a less sensitive marker of renal function in early diabetic nephropathy, but is frequently used along with SCr to evaluate patients on a day-to-day basis due to the ease of measurement.
- BUN is affected by a variety of conditions other than renal disease; despite these limitations, the BUN and SCr values remain useful, valid, and inexpensive measures of GFR.

Clinical Manifestations

1 Clinical manifestations of renal failure (Table 8.3) are evident when GFR is 20% to 35% of normal and patients become nephrotic with a urinary protein excretion >4 g/24 h. The clinical management of diabetes with nephrotic syndrome presents a great challenge. Management of glucose control becomes more difficult as loss of renal function diminishes renal catabolism of insulin, resulting in an increased half-life of the insulin.

Table 8.3. Clinical Manifestations of Renal Failure

Gastrointestinal	• Anorexia • Hiccups • Nausea, vomiting
Fluid and Electrolyte	• Fluid retention, weight gain • Electrolyte imbalance (ie, hyperkalemia)
Neuromuscular	• Fatigue • Muscle cramps • Changes in concentration, consciousness, behavior • Seizures • Coma • Asterixis
Cardiovascular and Pulmonary	• Congestive heart failure • Accelerated atherosclerosis • Pleural effusion
Hematologic and Immunologic	• Anemia • White blood cell count • Risk of bleeding • Risk of infection
Endocrine and Metabolic	• Increased risk for skeletal fractures • Osteomalacia • Altered calcium, phosphate metabolism

A Proteinuria is generally 4 to 8 g/24 h, but urinary protein loss can reach 20 to 30 g/24 h.

B Fluid retention is often massive, resulting in weight gain, peripheral edema, congestive heart failure, and pulmonary edema as uremia progresses.

- Fatigue and shortness of breath result in a reduction of daily activities.
- Hypertension may become uncontrolled secondary to fluid volume overload.

C Uremia becomes evident due to the accumulation of metabolic wastes and toxins.

- Anorexia, hiccups, nausea, and vomiting are gastrointestinal manifestations of uremia.
- Neuromuscular disturbances range in severity from early subtle changes in concentration, behavior, and level of consciousness to stupor, seizures, and coma.
- Anemia and its ensuing fatigue reflect the loss of renal synthesis of erythropoietin resulting in decreased red blood cell production. Other hematological and immunological abnormalities increase the risk of bleeding and infection.
- Renal osteodystrophy occurs due to impaired vitamin D metabolism and associated hypocalcemia resulting in secondary hyperparathyroidism.

2 Individuals with diabetic nephropathy appear to be more ill at equivalent levels of renal insufficiency than nondiabetic individuals. Underlying diabetes-induced neurological abnormalities, such as gastroparesis, can exacerbate uremia-induced nausea and vomiting.

Interventions for Patients With Diabetes at Risk of Renal Disease

1 Interventions are aimed at different stages of disease progression and include optimizing glycemic control, controlling blood pressure, and reducing dietary protein intake.

A Primary prevention strategies, such as optimizing glycemic control, may prevent the development of diabetic nephropathy.

B Secondary prevention strategies prevent or delay the progression from microalbuminuria to overt proteinuria.

- Aggressive control of blood pressure
- ACE inhibitor therapy
- Angiotensin II receptor blocker (ARB) therapy

C Tertiary prevention strategies may prevent or delay the progression of overt diabetic nephropathy and improve clinical outcomes. Tertiary care reduces morbidity and mortality by delaying time to dialysis or transplant.

2 The Diabetes Control and Complications Trial (DCCT)[39] and the United Kingdom Prospective Diabetes Study[42] demonstrated that maintaining strict glycemic control with intensive insulin and nutrition therapy delays the onset and slows the progression of early microvascular complications in patients with type 1 and type 2 diabetes.

3 Treatment for hypertension must be preceded by careful patient assessment.

A Assessment includes using the following questions to evaluate specific areas for intervention including weight; usual sodium, potassium, and alcohol intake; tobacco use; and activity pattern.

- At what weight are you most comfortable?

- What would have to happen in order for you to attain that weight?
- Have you noticed any swelling in your hands or your feet and legs?
- Does the swelling cause you any distress?
- Do you add salt to your food?
- Can you identify foods that you eat that are especially high in sodium?
- What are some ways that you can reduce your sodium intake?
- Do you use tobacco in any form? Have you ever considered quitting? What has to happen in order for you to reduce your tobacco consumption and eventually quit?
- We've talked about a lot of changes you'd like to make. On what are you most interested in working?

B Is the patient taking any drug (prescribed or over-the-counter) known to raise the blood pressure or glucose levels?

C Does the patient have a surgically correctable form of hypertension (renovascular disease or Cushing syndrome)?[68]

4 Antihypertensive drug therapy may slow the decline in renal function. However, all antihypertensive medications do not exert the same effect on the kidney in the presence of diabetes. ACE inhibitor therapy is considered as first-line therapy for all patients with diabetic nephropathy unless contraindications are present or side effects are intolerable.[69] In the case of side effects, an angiotensin II receptor blocker (ARB) may be an efficacious alternative.[70] Given the multisystem nature of diabetes, drug effects on renal function, metabolic control, and the cardiovascular and peripheral vascular systems must be considered.

A A single elevated blood pressure reading does not constitute a diagnosis of hypertension but indicates that additional observation is necessary.

B The primary hypertension goal for nonpregnant persons with diabetes and >18 years of age is to decrease blood pressure to and maintain it at <130 mmHg systolic and <85 mmHg diastolic.[1]

C Supine hypertension and orthostatic hypotension sometimes occur in patients with autonomic neuropathy. In this situation, it is recommended that blood pressure be determined supine, immediately on standing, and after 1 minute in the upright position.

D To help prevent extreme orthostatic reduction in blood pressure, the blood pressure in the standing position must be considered the therapeutic end point when evaluating treatment with antihypertensive agents.

E To establish timing and proper dosage of antihypertensive drugs, 24-hour ambulatory blood pressure recordings or home measurements can be obtained.
- Self-monitoring of blood pressure enhances educational efforts and allows the patient and the healthcare team to work together for detection, treatment, and evaluation.
- Reviewing patients' technique and checking blood pressure monitoring devices regularly can help ensure accurate readings.

F The initial pharmacological agent chosen is often an ACE inhibitor. Studies have demonstrated that ACE inhibitors given alone or with another antihypertensive agent produce a reduction in urinary albumin excretion rate.[37,38]

G Certain calcium antagonists have also demonstrated the ability to reduce microalbuminuria and proteinuria and therefore, theoretically, will reduce the progression of diabetic nephropathy.

- Some members of the dihydropyridine class of calcium channel blockers may increase urinary albumin excretion and should be avoided in patients with microalbuminuria and overt proteinuria.[71]
- Evidence also suggests that the use of calcium channel blockers may increase the risk of sudden death from acute myocardial infarction in patients with diabetes.[72]

H Loop diuretics, alpha-1 receptor blockers, thiazide diuretics in low dosages, and ß-blockers are all effective antihypertensive agents.

I Side effects can occur when using antihypertensive agents:
- Worsening of lipid levels and glycemic control from diuretics or ß-blockers
- Altered symptoms of hypoglycemia from ß-adrenergic blockers
- Fluid retention from sympathetic inhibitors, calcium channel blockers, and vasodilators
- Hyperkalemia and worsening azotemia when using an ACE inhibitor in patients with kidney disease

J Sodium restriction is also a central component of antihypertensive therapy.

5 The amount of protein in the diet affects renal size, structure, and function. Prospective studies have shown that in patients with type 1 diabetes with nephropathy, even moderate protein restriction resulted in a stabilization of renal function.[73,74] Studies also indicate vegetable protein may have less of an effect on hyperfiltration before nephropathy is diagnosed.[75] The role of a nutrition prescription containing <0.8 g protein/kg body weight remains controversial.

A The Recommended Dietary Allowance (RDA) for adults is an intake of 0.8 g protein/kg body weight.

B The usual dietary intake of protein in US diets is 1.2 to 1.4 g/kg of body weight/day.

C Almost all studies indicate renal benefit for even small reductions from usual amount of protein eaten (eg, achieved reduction to 0.8 to 1.0 g/kg body weight/day in individuals with microalbuminuria and 0.8 g/kg body weight/day or even possibly lower for individuals with clinical nephropathy).[76]

D This advice to reduce protein should be tempered with the need to maintain adequate nutritional status in patients with chronic renal failure before the development of ESRD.[76]

E Protein-restricted or other nutrient-altered pre-ESRD food/meal plans should be designed by a dietitian familiar with all components of medical nutrition therapy for diabetes.[76] The feasibility of long-term patient use of such restricted food/meal plans must be initially and continuously assessed by the dietitian and healthcare team.

F Use of protein-restricted meal plans can be assessed by measurement of urinary urea nitrogen (UUN). Patients using a protein-restricted meal plan must be continuously monitored for signs of malnutrition:
- Weight loss
- Muscle weakness
- Hypoalbuminemia

6 Preventive measures to reduce the risk of insult to the kidneys are recommended for patients with diabetes who are at risk for renal disease. Early identification and aggressive treatment of urinary tract infections are imperative to prevent further insult to the kidneys.

Table 8.4. Urinary Tract Infections

Patient Education	Guidelines for Health Professionals
• Teach patients about the signs and symptoms of a urinary tract infection	• Obtain cultures to detect specific organisms
• Teach patients to seek treatment right away if urgency, dysuria, or other signs of cystitis or a urinary tract infection occur	• Repeat urine cultures after treatment with antibiotics
• Teach female patients about emptying the bladder following sexual intercourse	• Determine whether bladder dysfunction is contributory
• Recommend consumption of cranberry juice, which acidifies the urine and has shown to reduce the incidence of urinary tract infections in elderly women	• Avoid placing an indwelling Foley catheter

A Guidelines for prevention and early treatment of urinary tract infections are listed in Table 8.4.

B Avoid nephrotoxic drugs.
  • If such agents (eg, aminoglycosides such as gentamicin) must be used, monitor blood levels and reduce the dosage of the drug administered to patients with impaired renal function.
  • Teach patients to use acetaminophen rather than nonsteroidal anti-inflammatory drugs because of the latter's effect of reducing prostaglandins.

C Avoid contrast dyes. If contrast media agents are necessary for tests, adequate hydration must be maintained before and after the study.

D Contrast media should not be administered to any person with diabetes whose serum creatinine level is >2 mg/dL (>265 µmol/L) unless the information sought is not available by any other means.

Choosing a Treatment Option for End-Stage Renal Disease

1 Treatments for ESRD are aimed at replacing the work of diseased kidneys. People with diabetes who receive transplants or dialysis experience higher morbidity and mortality than patients without diabetes because of coexisting complications such as coronary artery disease, retinopathy, and neuropathy. Providing education and information on each treatment option allows the patient and family to make an informed choice and enhances the chances for a positive outcome.

  A Benefits and risks of each treatment option should be reviewed with patients and family members for a comparison of options in uremia therapy (Table 8.5).[77]

  B Direct contact with other patients who are receiving different forms of therapy for ESRD may be valuable for education, emotional support, and instilling hope.

  C Common medications used when treating ESRD include[78]

Table 8.5. Comparison of Uremia Treatment Options for Patients With Diabetes and End-Stage Renal Disease

	Renal Transplantation	CAPD	Home Hemodialysis
Advantages	• Permits long intervals away from treatment facility • Best rehabilitation • Reverses uremic state completely • Patient survival often >10 y	• Avoids major surgery • Minimizes cardiovascular stress (volume shifts) • Facilitates glucose control (when insulin added to dialysate) • Can be readily taught for home dialysis • No need for vascular access	• Avoids major surgery • Type 2 patients have survived >10 yr • rHuEPO* may improve rehabilitation
Disadvantages	• Steroids exacerbate poor metabolic control • Cyclosporine exacerbates hypertension • Risk of infection • Inability to predict risk of diabetes in familial donors • May not be appropriate in severe cardiovascular disease, chronically infected patients • Risk of recurrent diabetic nephropathy • Retinopathy progresses in 30% of patients	• High technique failure rate, mortality • Risk of peritonitis • Retinopathy progresses • Risk of patient burnout from daily repetitive nature of technique	• Requires committed partner • "Failure-to-thrive" in about one third of patients • Mortality similar to cadaveric kidney recipients • Retinopathy progresses • Requires vascular access

*rHuEPO = recombinant human erythropoietin
Source: Adapted from Markell and Friedman.[7]

- Multivitamins or vitamins B and C are taken to replace those vitamins lost in dialysis.
- Calcium citrate is used to prevent renal bone disease or renal osteodystrophy. Calcium is usually taken with meals to bind the phosphorous, but it can also be taken without regard to meals to raise the calcium level in the body.
- Calcitriol (1α,25-dihydroxycholecalciferol) may be prescribed to help improve absorption of calcium. It is the most potent form of vitamin D available.
- Ferrous sulfate is taken to restore iron stores depleted by anemia or administration of erythropoietin therapy. Iron supplements should be taken separately from calcium carbonate (phosphorous binders) to improve absorption.
- Epoetin alpha (EPO) is given to correct anemia associated with ESRD. It is given subcutaneously or intravenously to increase the hematocrit.

2 Planning for treatment should begin early, usually when the serum creatinine level reaches 3 mg/dL (265 µmol/L).

A Planning includes tissue typing of family members for possible kidney transplant donation, being placed on a cadaveric waiting list, and/or creating vascular access for dialysis.

B Circumstances may exist that limit the patient's choice of treatment. For example, those with cardiovascular disease or vascular access problems might be less suitable candidates for hemodialysis, or those unable to tolerate fluid in the peritoneal cavity would not be appropriate candidates for peritoneal dialysis.

Treatment Options for End-Stage Renal Disease

1 No treatment.

A If no treatment is administered, death will result usually within 7 months. This option is an elective decision for some patients.

B The patient and family should consider the no-treatment option after the patient is dialyzed and nonuremic because of uremia's effect on mental status.

C Encourage the patient and family to discuss this decision with clergy, a psychologist, a social worker, the healthcare team, and other family members.

D Planning supportive care (eg, home care, hospice care) is necessary for the patient who wishes to forego treatment.

2 Hemodialysis is a process of cleansing or filtering the blood of nitrogenous wastes. The patient's blood is circulated and cleansed outside of the body. With effective dialysis treatments, uremia can be treated and the patient can achieve an improved level of health and well-being, including a vigorous appetite. The following hemodialysis process and factors should be considered.

A The filter used for hemodialysis is a semipermeable membrane. This membrane is a thin material with holes that permits the passage of small particles but retains larger particles.

B During dialysis, the patient's blood passes on one side of the membrane, while dialysate (prepared dialysis solution) passes on the other side of the membrane. The solution removes fluid and particles (waste products) from the blood by diffusive clearance.

C Blood is withdrawn through a needle inserted in a specially prepared blood vessel, usually a synthetic graft or an arteriovenous fistula (using the patient's own blood vessels) located in the patient's forearm. The needle is attached by plastic tubing to a hemodialysis machine. A pump keeps blood moving through the dialyzer as wastes and fluid are filtered out. The cleansed blood returns to the patient through another needle in the same or an adjacent blood vessel.

D Hemodialysis can be performed in an ambulatory setting or in the patient's home. Treatments are usually given 3 times per week and take 3 to 6 hours to complete.

E Because the blood is not being cleansed 24 hours a day, the patient must still use an individualized renal food/meal plan with fluid restriction.

F Treatment of the associated anemia has a significant effect on rehabilitation in this population, improving quality-of-life indicators and employment status.[79]

G Patients with diabetes receiving dialytic therapy might be oliguric and therefore not experience the osmotic diuresis that typically accompanies hyperglycemia in a patient with diabetes not undergoing dialysis. Satisfying the thirst that accompanies hyperglycemia might be an additional challenge for the patient while on a fluid-restricted diet.[69] Chewing gum or sucking on hard candy or lemon wedges may help.

H Factors that can alter glucose levels for the patient receiving hemodialysis treatment include the glucose concentration in the dialysate bath, appetite alteration on dialysis days and "off" days, decreased activity on dialysis days, and emotional stress.

I The following questions can be used to help elicit information regarding causes of blood glucose variability in patients with diabetes who are receiving hemodialysis treatments:

- What is your glucose pattern on days you are having dialysis?
- What is your pattern on other days?
- When (and how much) do you eat on days you are having dialysis?
- What about other days?
- What is your activity pattern like on days you are having dialysis?
- What is your activity pattern on other days?
- What is your hematocrit?
- What is the acceptable hematocrit range for the meter you are using?
- On a scale of 1 to 10, with 1 being very low and 10 being very high, how would you rate your level of stress on dialysis days? How does this compare to other days?

J Sometimes a change in the type of glucose meter used may be warranted to avoid measuring erroneous blood glucose values. Meter manufacturers provide specifications of hematocrit ranges for their meters (see Chapter 4, Monitoring, Diabetes Management Therapies, for more information).

3 Peritoneal dialysis takes place inside the body by employing the body's own capillary and serosal membranes.

A Blood is filtered through the peritoneal membrane that lines the abdominal cavity.

- Surgery is required to place a catheter through an opening in the wall of the abdominal cavity. This opening is needed so that the dialysis solution can be instilled into the peritoneal cavity and waste products can pass from the bloodstream into the dialysis solution.
- The used solution is drained and replaced with a new solution on a regular basis.

B Currently, 3 types of peritoneal dialysis are being used.

- *Continuous ambulatory peritoneal dialysis (CAPD)* is a manual method of performing peritoneal dialysis. The patient exchanges new fluid (dialysate) every 4 to 6 hours during a 24-hour period each day. The dialysate passes from a plastic bag through the catheter and stays in the patient's abdomen with the catheter sealed. The dialysate is drained after several hours, then the process begins again with fresh dialysate solution.
- *Continuous cyclic peritoneal dialysis (CCPD)* is like CAPD except a machine that is connected to the catheter automatically fills and drains the dialysate solution from the patient's abdomen. This type of dialysis can be performed at night while the patient is sleeping. Assistance from a family member, friend, or health professional is needed to perform CCPD.
- *Intermittent peritoneal dialysis (IPD)* uses the same type of machine as CCPD to fill and drain the dialysate solution from the patient's abdomen. IPD treatments take longer than CCPD, and assistance is needed from a family member, friend, or health professional.

C Patients requiring insulin can administer regular insulin directly into the dialysate before the dialysate is instilled into the peritoneal cavity. Intraperitoneal insulin regimen has the following advantages:

- Provides a continuous insulin infusion.
- Eliminates the need for injections.
- May provide a more physiologic route of absorption, since the exogenous insulin is absorbed into the portal vein, which mimics the action of pancreatic insulin.

D Intraperitoneal insulin has the following disadvantages:

- Provides an additional source of bacterial contamination for the dialysate during injection of insulin into the bags.
- Results in higher total insulin doses due to loss of spent dialysate.

E Regular insulin works to metabolize the dietary glucose that is consumed as well as the highly concentrated dextrose in the dialysate solution. Table 8.6 outlines insulin adjustments for dialysis.[80]

F Visually impaired and blind patients have been successful in performing peritoneal dialysis.

G Factors that can affect glucose regulation for patients on peritoneal dialysis include the concentration of the dialysate solution, method(s) of insulin delivery (eg, intraperitoneal, subcutaneous, or both), and infection (peritonitis).

H The following questions can be used to help assess factors that may contribute to variability in blood glucose levels.

- What is the dextrose concentration of the solution you are using for your peritoneal dialysis: 1.5%, 2.5%, or 4.25%?
- What type(s) of insulin are you using?
- When are you taking your insulin?
- Where on your body are you injecting the insulin?
- Are there any signs of infection (catheter-related or peritonitis)?

4 Kidney transplantation can be performed using a kidney from a living related donor, a living unrelated donor, or a suitable cadaveric donor.

Table 8.6. Insulin Adjustments for Patients on CAPD or CCPD

Concentration of Glucose in Dialysate (g/dL)	Additional Insulin in Units/Liter of Dialysate Solution
0.005	0
1.5	1
2.5	2
4.25	3

Fasting Blood Glucose	1 Hour Post-Prandial Glucose	Change in Baseline Insulin in Units/2 Liters of Dialysate Solution
—	<40 mg/dL	-6 units
<40 mg/dL	40 mg/dL	-4 units
40 mg/dL	80 mg/dL	-2 units
80 to 140 mg/dL	120 to 180 mg/dL	No change
180 mg/dL	240 mg/dL	+2 units
240 mg/dL	>240 mg/dL	+4 units
>240 mg/dL		+6 units or more May need additional subq

Source: Reprinted with permission from Tzamaloukas.[80]

A Once transplantation has occurred, immunosuppressive medications are required throughout the patient's life to prevent the body from rejecting the transplanted organ.

B Patients with diabetes must take additional insulin following transplantation because the newly functioning kidney catabolizes insulin once again, posttransplant steroid therapy has a hyperglycemic effect, and the patient experiences a notable increase in appetite, which can lead to weight gain.

C Following transplantation, blood glucose control may be altered by the following factors:
- Degree of function of the transplanted kidney
- Treatment for transplant rejection
- Changes in steroid dose
- Patient's increased appetite and ability to consume a more liberal diet with subsequent weight gain
- Diuretic therapy
- Presence of infection (transplant patients are more susceptible to infection because of immunosuppression)

D The following questions can be used to help detect the cause of variability in blood glucose levels:

- What is your current immunosuppression regimen?
- Does that regimen represent an increase or decrease from your usual dose of immunosuppressive medication?
- How much weight have you gained since your transplant?
- Are you being treated for any infection?
- What antihypertensive/diuretic agents are you currently taking?
- What is your current exercise/activity schedule?

5 Patients with type 1 diabetes may be considered for a simultaneous kidney-pancreas transplantation.

A A kidney-pancreas transplantation restores both glucose metabolism and kidney function.

B Criteria for patient selection vary at each transplant center but typically include the following:
- Diagnosis of type 1 diabetes
- Evidence of secondary complications such as renal insufficiency or preproliferative retinopathy
- Metabolic instability
- Adequate financial resources/insurance coverage (insurance carriers review eligibility for payment on a case-by-case basis)

C Contraindications for kidney-pancreas transplantation include
- Presence of HIV
- Malignancy
- Psychosis
- Any active infection
- Severe neuropathies
- Inoperable cardiovascular disease

D Complications of kidney-pancreas transplantation include
- Cardiac incompetence
- Arterial or venous thrombosis
- Anastomotic leaks, bleeding
- Side effects of immunosuppression (Table 8.7)[81]
- Pancreatitis
- Metabolic acidosis related to exocrine pancreatic function

E Transplantation can be justified if the complications of diabetes are more dangerous than the side effects of immunosuppression.

F Renal transplant function is easier to measure than pancreas function.
- A rise in serum creatinine is a primary indicator of kidney rejection.
- A decrease in urinary amylase production can signal a pancreas in jeopardy.
- Hyperglycemia occurs late in pancreas rejection.
- Signs of rejection can be detected earlier in the kidney and treatment can be initiated, thus providing some protection for the pancreas.
- Living related donors must be screened carefully because of their risk for developing diabetes. Brain-dead cadavers are a more common donor source.[81,82]

Table 8.7. Side Effects of Immunosuppression

Prednisone	• Sodium, water retention • Increased appetite • Increased fat deposits • Hyperkalemia • Muscle wasting • Increased serum cholesterol • Calcium loss • Sun sensitivity • Mood swings	• Increased stomach acid • Night sweats • Increased hair • Acne • Blurred vision • Slowed healing • Muscle weakness • Susceptibility to infection
Cyclosporine	• Flushing • Hair growth • Fine tremor • Gingival hyperplasia • Paresthesias • Hypertension • Gastrointestinal distress • Nephrotoxicity	
Sulfa drugs	• Liver toxicity • Decreased leukocytes • Allergy • Sun sensitivity • Gastrointestinal symptoms • Renal toxicity	
Azathioprine	• Decreased leukocytes • Liver toxicity • Hair loss • Allergy	
Antacid drugs	• Diarrhea or constipation • Low phosphorous • High magnesium	
Antilymphocyte globin	• Allergy • Decreased leukocytes • Decreased platelets	

Source: Adapted from Nettles.[81]

Psychosocial Issues in End-Stage Renal Disease

1 Rates of depression, anxiety, and stress may be higher among dialysis patients than among the general population. These psychological reactions may occur in response to the losses associated with diabetes and renal disease (eg, loss of physical capacities and loss of control from the complications associated with diabetes).

2 Patients respond in a variety of ways to receiving a diagnosis of renal disease. Some typical responses include:

A "No one ever told me this could happen."

B "My life is over."

C "It's all my fault, if only I had taken better care of myself."

D "It's all my doctor's fault."

E "I feel like my body is falling apart, piece by piece."

3 It is imperative to assess and comprehend how each patient and family respond to the patient's illness.

A A variety of healthcare professionals, including mental health professionals, need to be involved in helping patients and families adjust to their losses and to a new, often complex treatment regimen.[83]

B Some patients blame themselves when they develop complications of diabetes.

C Scare tactics (eg, "If you don't control your blood glucose, you will go into kidney failure.") are not an effective behavior change strategy.

D Avoid giving "pat" answers or responses which can sound patronizing. By asking "would it help to know that complications such as diabetic nephropathy can develop in patients who have done their best to maintain optimal glucose control," the healthcare team can communicate this possibility to the patient and family and perhaps help lessen the feelings of guilt and blame that can occur with a diagnosis of ESRD.

4 An effective intervention for some patients with ESRD is to invite them to join a support group or to pair new patients with patients who have had success using one of the various renal replacement therapies.

A Patients can learn new information, coping skills and behaviors, and positive attitudes from these role models.

B Patients, their families, and the healthcare team can benefit from having members from a support group available in the clinic setting to meet with new patients who face a diagnosis of renal disease.

Self-Review Questions

1 What is the annual cost of treatment for ESRD in the US in patients with diabetes?

2 Define creatinine clearance, BUN, and nephrotic syndrome.

3 State 4 of the 7 functions of the kidney.

4 What percentage of people with type 1 diabetes develop renal failure?

5 What percentage of people with type 2 diabetes develop renal failure?

6 Describe the progression of renal disease in patients with type 1 diabetes.

7 Identify 4 risk factors for diabetic nephropathy.

8 Identify the laboratory tests used most frequently to diagnose diabetic nephropathy and monitor renal function.

9 Name the first clinical sign indicative of kidney damage for a person with diabetes and how often an assessment should be conducted.

10 List the clinical manifestations of diabetic kidney disease.

11 Describe interventions used to prevent or slow the progression of diabetic nephropathy.

12 Describe potential food/nutrition modifications that may be needed at different stages of diabetic nephropathy.

13 Name factors that can harm the kidneys, and describe how these factors can be minimized.

14 Describe treatment options for ESRD and their impact on diabetes management.

15 Contrast microalbuminuria with proteinuria.

Learning Assessment: Case Study 1

MB is a 53-year-old engineer who is married and is the mother of 3 grown children. She has been referred because of an elevated HbA1c despite taking a combination of glyburide 20 mg and metformin 1500 mg daily. The only other medication she takes is hydrochlorothiazide 25 mg daily. She is familiar with SMBG but stopped testing because her glucose was always high. She denies a previous history of known complications from diabetes. MB is of normal weight, her blood pressure is 130/98 mmHg with no postural change, and both fundi show moderate background retinopathy. She has trace pedal edema and mild stocking-glove sensory deficit in both lower extremities. Laboratory results show a BUN of 32, creatinine of 2.4, potassium of 4.3, 24-hour urine protein excretion of 945 mg, and creatinine clearance of 38 mL/min. Her HbA1c is 9.8% (normal = 3.4% to 6.2%). After reviewing the answers to MB's diabetes knowledge and self-care questionnaire, you determine she demonstrates a lack of knowledge about both diabetes management and kidney disease.

Questions for Discussion

1 What teaching plan would you develop with MB and how would you begin?

2 What interventions could the healthcare team employ immediately?

3 What are potential psychosocial issues for this patient?

Discussion

1 A priority at this first visit is to begin to establish rapport and a relationship between MB and the other key members of the healthcare team.

A Team members should meet with MB over the next few weeks in order to individually assess her needs and desired level of involvement in her care. This time is an opportunity for MB to identify specific goals toward which she would like to work. These visits give the educator the opportunity to provide information to MB and allow for discussion regarding the importance of her role in her care.

B Initiate regular visits and telephone contact to answer questions and reinforce MB's desired behavior change.

C Review MB's SMBG technique. Her feelings and concerns regarding SMBG also need to be explored.

D Ask what would make SMBG relevant for her and discuss how often she believes she needs to test to reach her blood glucose goals.

E Assist MB in learning how to use the information she obtains through SMBG.

F Let MB know that this can be her opportunity to take charge of her diabetes which may help to slow the progression of kidney damage.

G Offer MB and her family introductory information on kidney disease, including function, preventive measures, terminology, and what tests are used to track kidney function and how often they are needed.

H Preventive measures related to eye and foot care must be reviewed and reinforced. The educator can use the time during MB's foot exam to stress the importance of daily self-inspection of shoes and feet.

2 Interventions that could be employed include

A Metformin should be discontinued immediately; this medication is contraindicated in patients with an elevated serum creatinine due to increased risk of lactic acidosis.

B If MB expresses a desire to improve her glucose control, review options for optimizing glycemic control.

C If MB is agreeable, insulin therapy should be initiated.

D Blood pressure control must be achieved. The addition of an ACE inhibitor to her current diuretic therapy is warranted. This medication may not only reduce her blood pressure, but the level of proteinuria may also be decreased.

• Discuss the benefits of a lower blood pressure on her kidney function and the value of frequent blood pressure measurement. MB may be interested in monitoring the effects of her sodium intake and the addition of the ACE inhibitor on her daily blood pressure.

• Options for frequent blood pressure measurements include obtaining a blood pressure monitor for home use.

E Because MB is at risk for hyperkalemia with the addition of the ACE inhibitor, she will need a review of the usual sources of potassium-rich foods in her diet.

F Decreasing sodium may eliminate her pedal edema.

G Provide a referral to the ophthalmologist for a baseline retinal examination and develop a treatment plan to further evaluate for MB's moderate background retinopathy.

3 Potential psychosocial issues for MB include

A The emotional impact of the diagnosis of kidney damage.

• MB and her family will need support from the healthcare team with time allotted to discuss fears and concerns related to the diagnosis.

• A referral to a psychologist or a social worker may help MB explore her feelings and coping ability concerning the diagnosis of kidney disease and identify sources of emotional and financial support.

B Given changes in diabetes and hypertension management, new medications, and the amount of education needed, the educator can work with MB to prioritize her teaching, according to MB's stated goals.

C The educator should be available to MB by telephone and should schedule a series of return visits to answer questions and provide further information, support, or referral.

D Although renal replacement therapy is not currently indicated, when MB displays readiness and asks about the treatment for ESRD, a discussion regarding her options for renal replacement therapy should be initiated.

References

1   American Diabetes Association. Diabetic nephropathy (position statement). Diabetes Care. 2001;24(suppl 1):S69-S72.

2   Herman W, Hawthorne V, Hamman R, Keen H, et al. Consensus statement. Am J Kidney Dis. 1989;13(1):2-6.

3   Deckert T, Poulsen JE, Larsen M. Prognosis of diabetics with diabetes onset before the age of thirty-one. I. Survival, causes of death, and complications. Diabetologia. 1978;14:363-370.

4   Dorman JS, LaPorte RE, Kuller LH, et al. The Pittsburgh Insulin-dependent Diabetes Mellitus (IDDM) Morbidity and Mortality Study. Mortality results. Diabetes. 1984;33:271-276.

5   Andersen AR, Christiansen, JS, Andersen JK, Kreiner S, Deckert T. Diabetic nephropathy in Type 1 (insulin-dependent) diabetes: an epidemiologic study. Diabetologia. 1983;25:496-501.

6   Borch-Johnsen K, Andersen PK, Deckert T. The effect of proteinuria on relative mortality in Type 1 (insulin-dependent) diabetes mellitus. Diabetologia. 1985;28:590-596.

7   Jensen T, Borch-Johnsen K, Kofoed-Enevoldsen A, Deckert T. Coronary heart disease in young Type 1 (insulin-dependent) diabetic patients with and without diabetic nephropathy: incidence and risk factors. Diabetologia. 1987; 30:144-148.

8   Krolewski AS, Kosinski EJ, Warram JH, et al. Magnitude and determinants of coronary artery disease in juvenile-onset, insulin-dependent diabetes mellitus. Am J Cardiol. 1987;59:750-755.

9   Borch-Johnsen K, Kreiner S. Proteinuria: value as predictor of cardiovascular mortality in insulin dependent diabetes mellitus. Br Med J. 1987;294:1651-1654.

10 Rettig BS, Teutsch SM. The incidence of end-stage renal disease in Type I and Type II diabetes mellitus. Diabetic Nephropathy. 1984;3:26-27.

11 Cowie CC, Port FK, Wolfe RA, Savage PJ, Moll PP, Hawthorne VM. Disparities in incidence of diabetic end-stage renal disease according to race and type of diabetes. N Engl J Med. 1989;321:1074-1079.

12 Mogensen CE, Chachati A, Christensen CK, et al. Microalbuminuria: an early marker of renal involvement in diabetes. Uremia Invest. 1985;9:85-95.

13 Mogensen CE. Urinary albumin excretion in early and long-term juvenile diabetes. Scand J Clin Lab Invest. 1971;28:183-193.

14 Feldt-Rasmussen B, Mathiesen ER. Variability of urinary albumin excretion in incipient diabetic nephropathy. Diabetic Nephropathy. 1984;3:101-103.

15 Feldt-Rasmussen B, Dinesen B, Deckert M. Enzyme immunoassay: an improved determination of urinary albumin in diabetics with incipient nephropathy. Scand J Clin Lab Invest. 1985;45:539-544.

16 Cowell CT, Rogers S, Silink M. First morning urinary albumin concentration is a good predictor of 24-hour urinary albumin excretion in children with Type 1 (insulin-dependent) diabetes. Diabetologia. 1986;29:97-99.

17 Cohen DL, Close CF, Viberti GC. The variability of overnight urinary albumin excretion in insulin-dependent diabetic and normal subjects. Diabetic Medicine. 1987;4:437-440.

18 Ellis D, Coonrod BA, Dorman JS, Kelsey SF, Becker DJ, Avner ED, Orchard TJ: Choice of urine sample predictive of microalbuminuria in patients with insulin-dependent diabetes mellitus. Am J Kidney Dis. 1989;13:321-328.

19 National Institute of Diabetes and Digestive and Kidney Diseases. US Renal Data Systems (USRDS) 1996 Annual Report. Bethesda, Md: National Institute of Diabetes and Digestive and Kidney Diseases; 1996:April.

20 DeFronzo RA. Diabetic nephropathy. In: Therapy for Diabetes Mellitus and Related Disorders. 3rd ed. Lebovitz HE, ed. Alexandria, Va: American Diabetes Association; 1998:338-363.

21 DeFronzo RA. Diabetic nephropathy: etiologic and therapeutic considerations. Diabetes Reviews. 1995;3:510-564.

22 Brancati, FL, Whittle JC, Whelton PK, Seidler AJ, Kiag MJ. The excess incidence of diabetic end-stage renal disease among blacks: a population-based study of potential explanatory factors. JAMA. 1992;268:3079-3084.

23 Mogensen CE, Christensen CK, Vittinghus E. The stages in diabetic renal disease with emphasis on the stage of incipient diabetic nephropathy. Diabetes. 1983;32(suppl 2):64-78.

24 Selby JV, FitzSimmons SC, Newman JM, et al. The natural history and epidemiology of diabetic nephropathy. Implications for prevention and control. JAMA. 1990;263:1954-1960.

25 Mogensen CE, Christensen CK. Predicting diabetic nephropathy in insulin-dependent patients. N Engl J Med. 1984;311:89-93.

26 Viberti GC, Hill RD, Jarrett RJ, Argyropoulos A, Mahmud U, Keen H. Microalbuminuria as a predictor of clinical nephropathy in insulin-dependent diabetes mellitus. Lancet. 1982;I:1430-1432.

27 Parving H-H, Oxenboll B, Svendsen PA, Sandahl Christiansen J, Andersen AR. Early detection of patients at risk of developing diabetic nephropathy. A longitudinal study of urinary albumin excretion. Acta Endocrinol. 1982;100:550-555.

28 Mathiesen ER, Oxenboll B, Johnsen K, Svendsen PA, Deckert T. Incipient nephropathy in Type 1 (insulin-dependent) diabetes. Diabetologia. 1984;26:406-410.

29 Mogensen CE. Microalbuminuria predicts clinical proteinuria and early mortality in maturity-onset diabetes. N Engl J Med. 1984;310:356-360.

30 Jarrett RJ, Viberti GC, Argyropoulos A, Hill RD, Mahmud U, Murrells TJ. Microalbuminuria predicts mortality in non-insulin-dependent diabetes. Diabetic Medicine. 1984;1:17-19.

31 Lewis EJ, Hunsicker LG, Bain RP, Rhode RD. The effect of angiotensin-converting-enzyme inhibition on diabetic nephropathy. N Engl J Med. 1993;329:1456-1462.

32 Tuttle KR, DeFronzo RA, Stein JH. Treatment of diabetic nephropathy: a rational approach based on its pathophysiology. Semin Nephrol. 1991;11:220-235.

33 Castellino P, Shohat J, DeFronzo RA. Hyperfiltration and diabetic nephropathy: is it the beginning? Or is it the end? Semin Nephrol. 1990;10:228-241.

34 Franz MJ. Protein controversies in diabetes. Diabetes Spectrum. 2000;13:132-141.

35 Marcus AO. Diabetes mellitus: nephropathy and hypertension. Clin Diabetes. 1996;14:91-94.

36 Savage S, Nagel NJ, Estacio RO, Lukken N, Schrier RW. Clinical factors associated with urinary albumin excretion in type 2 diabetes. Am J Kidney Dis. 1995;25:836-844.

37 Ravid M, Lang R, Rachmani R, Lishner M. Long-term renoprotective effect of angiotensin-converting enzyme inhibition in non-insulin-dependent diabetes mellitus: a 7-year follow-up study. Arch Intern Med. 1996;156:286-289.

38 Ravid M, Savin H, Jutrin I, Bental T, Katz B, Lishner M. Long-term stabilizing effect of angiotensin-converting enzyme inhibition on plasma creatinine and on proteinuria in normotensive type 2 diabetic patients. Ann Intern Med. 1993;118:577-581.

39 The Diabetes Control and Complications Trial Research Group. The effect of intensive treatment of diabetes on the development and progression of long-term complications in insulin-dependent diabetes. N Engl J Med. 1993;329:977-986.

40 Reichard P, Nilsson BY, Rosenqvist U. The effect of long-term intensified insulin treatment on the development of microvascular complications of diabetes mellitus. N Engl J Med. 1993;329:304-309.

41 Ohkubo Y, Kishikawa H, Araki E, et al. Intensive insulin therapy prevents the progression of diabetic microvascular complications in Japanese patients with non-insulin dependent diabetes mellitus: a randomized prospective 6-year study. Diabetes Research and Clinical Practice. 1995;28:103-117.

42 UK Prospective Diabetes Study (UKPDS) Group. Intensive blood-glucose control with sulphonylureas or insulin compared with conventional treatment and risk of complications in patients with type 2 diabetes (UKPDS 33). Lancet. 1998;352:837-853.

43 Nyberg G, Norden G, Attman P-O, et al. Diabetic nephropathy: is dietary protein harmful? Diabetic Complications. 1987;1:37-40.

44 Watts GF, Gregory L, Naoumova R, Kubal C, Shaw KM. Nutrient intake in insulin-dependent diabetic patients with incipient nephropathy. Eur J Clin Nutr. 1988;42:697-702.

45 Ekberg G, Sjofors G, Grefberg N, Larsson L-O, Vaara I. Protein intake and glomerular hyperfiltration in insulin-treated diabetic without manifest nephropathy. Scan J Urol Nephrol. 1993;27:441-446.

46 Jameel N, Pugh JA, Mitchell BD, Stern MP. Dietary protein is not correlated with clinical proteinuria in NIDDM. Diabetes Care. 1992;15:178-183.

47 Riley MD, Dwyer T. Microalbuminuria is positively associated with usual dietary saturated fat intake and negatively associated with usual protein intake in people with insulin-dependent diabetes mellitus. Am J Clin Nutr. 1998;67:50-57.

48 Toeller M, Buyken A, Heitkamp G, et al, and the EURODIAB IDDM Complications Study Group. Protein intake and urinary albumin excretion rates in EURODIAB IDDM Complications Study. Diabetologia. 1997;40:1219-1226.

49 Christiansen JS. Cigarette smoking and prevalence of microangiopathy in juvenile-onset insulin-dependent diabetes mellitus. Diabetes Care. 1978;1:146-149.

50 Telmer S, Sandahl Christiansen J, Andersen AR, Nerup J, Deckert T. Smoking habits and prevalence of clinical diabetic microangiopathy in insulin-dependent diabetics. Acta Med Scand. 1984;215:63-68.

51 Norden G, Nyberg G. Smoking and diabetic nephropathy. Acta Med Scand. 1984;215:257-261.

52 Muhlhauser I, Sawicki P, Berger M. Cigarette-smoking as a risk factor for macroproteinuria and proliferative retinopathy in Type 1 (insulin-dependent) diabetes. Diabetologia. 1986;29:500-502.

53 Orchard TJ, Dorman JS, Maser RE, et al. Prevalence of complications in IDDM by sex and duration. Pittsburgh Epidemiology of Diabetes Complications Study II. Diabetes. 1990;39:1116-1124.

54 Kofoed-Enevoldsen A, Borch-Johnsen K, Kreiner S, Nerup J, Deckert T: Declining incidence of persistent proteinuria in Type I (insulin-dependent) diabetic patients in Denmark. Diabetes. 1987;36:205-209.

55 Herman WH, Teutsch SM. Kidney diseases associated with diabetes. In Diabetes in America. Diabetes Data Compiled 1984. National Diabetes Data Group. US Department of Health and Human Services, Public Health Service, National Institutes of Health, National Institute of Arthritis, Diabetes, and Digestive and Kidney Diseases; 1985, NIH 85-1468:XIV1-31.

56 Pugh JA. The epidemiology of diabetic nephropathy. Diabetes Metab Rev. 1989;5:531-545.

57 Hasslacher C, Stech W, Wahl P, Ritz E. Blood pressure and metabolic control as risk factors for nephropathy in Type 1 (insulin-dependent) diabetes. Diabetologia. 1985;28:6-11.

58 Klein R, Klein BEK, Moss SE, Davis MD, DeMets DL. The Wisconsin Epidemiologic Study of Diabetes Retinopathy: V. Proteinuria and retinopathy in a population of diabetic persons diagnosed prior to 30 years of age. In: Diabetic Renal-Retinal Syndrome. Vol. 3. Friedman EA, L'Esperance FA Jr, eds. Orlando, Fl: Grune & Stratton; 1986:245-264.

59 Viberti GC, Keen H, Wiseman MJ. Raised arterial pressure in parents of proteinuric insulin dependent diabetics. Br Med J. 1987;295:515-517.

60 Krolewski AS, Canessa M, Warram JH, et al. Predisposition to hypertension and susceptibility to renal disease in insulin-dependent diabetes mellitus. N Engl J Med. 1988;318:140-145.

61 Hamilton M, Pickering GW, Roberts JAF, Sowry GSC. The aetiology of essential hypertension. 4. The role of inheritance. Clin Sci. 1954;13:273-304.

62 Hayes CG, Tyroler HA, Cassel JC. Family aggregation of blood pressure in Evans County, Georgia. Arch Intern Med. 1971;128:965-975.

63 Stamler R, Stamler J, Riedlinger WF, Algera G, Roberts RH. Family (parental) history and prevalence of hypertension. Results of a nationwide screening program. JAMA. 1979;241:34-36.

64 Munger RG, Prineas RJ, Gomez-Marin O. Persistent elevation of blood pressure among children with a family history of hypertension: the Minneapolis children's blood pressure study. J Hypertens. 1988;6:647-653.

65 Seaquist ER, Goetz FC, Rich S, Barbosa J. Familial clustering of diabetic kidney disease. Evidence for genetic susceptibility to diabetic nephropathy. N Engl J Med. 1989;320:1161-1165.

66 Borch-Johnsen K, Norgaard K, Jensen JS, Deckert T. Diabetic nephropathy—an inherited complication? Diabetes. 1990;39(suppl 1):71A.

67 Carlson JA, Harrington JT. Laboratory evaluation of renal function. In: Diseases of the Kidney. 5th ed. Schrier RW, Gottschalk CW, eds. Boston: Little & Brown; 1993:361-405.

68 National High Blood Pressure Education Program Working Group. Report on hypertension and chronic renal failure. Arch Intern Med; 1991;151:1280-1287.

69 Vijan S, Stevens DL, Herman WH, Funnell MM, Standiford CJ. Screening, prevention, counseling, and treatment for the complications of type 2 diabetes mellitus. J Gen Intern Med. 1997;12:567-580.

70 Lacourciere Y, Belanger A, Godin C, et al. Long-term comparison of losartan and enalapril on kidney function in hypertensive type 2 diabetics with early nephropathy. Kidney Int. 2000;58:762-769.

71 Abbott K, Smith A, Bakris G. Effects of dihydropyridine calcium antagonists on albuminuria in patients with diabetes. J Clin Pharmacol. 1996;36:274-279.

72 Estacio R, Jeffers, B, Hiatt, W, et al. The effect of nisoldipine as compared with enalapril on cardiovascular outcome inpatients with non-insulin-dependent diabetes and hypertension. N Engl J Med. 1998;338:645-652.

73 Zeller K, Whittaker E, Sullivan L, Raskin P, Jacobson HR. Effect of restricting dietary protein on the progression of renal failure in patients with insulin-dependent diabetes mellitus. N Engl J Med. 1991;324:78-84.

74 Pedrini MT, Levey AS, Lau J, Chalmers TC, Wang PH. The effect of dietary protein restriction on the progression of diabetic and nondiabetic renal diseases: a meta-analysis. Ann Intern Med. 1996;124:627-632.

75 Wheeler ML. Nephropathy and medical nutrition therapy. In: American Diabetes Association Guide to Medical Nutrition Therapy for Diabetes. Franz MJ, Bantle JP, eds. Alexandria, Va: American Diabetes Association; 1999:312-329.

76 Franz MJ, Bantle JP, Beebe CA, et al. Evidence-based nutrition principles and recommendations for diabetes and related complications (technical review). Diabetes Care. In press.

77 Markell MS, Friedman EA. Care of the diabetic patient with end-stage renal disease. Semin Nephrol. 1990;10:274-286.

78 Kleinbeck C. Challenges of diabetes and dialysis. Diabetes Spectrum. 1997;10:135-141.

79 Delano BG. Improvements in quality of life following treatment with rHuEPO in anemic hemodialysis patients. Am J Kidney Dis. 1989;14(suppl 1):14-18.

80 Tzamaloukas AH. Diabetes. In: Handbook of Dialysis. 2nd ed. Daugirdas JT, Ing TS, eds. Boston: Little & Brown; 1994:422-432.

81 Nettles AT. Pancreas transplantation: a University of Minnesota perspective. Diabetes Educ. 1992;18:232-238.

82 Trusler LA. Simultaneous kidney-pancreas transplantation. ANNA J. 1991;18:487-491.

83 Kopp J. Psychosocial correlates of diabetes and renal dysfunction. ANNA J. 1992;19:432-437.

Suggested Readings

Alzaid AA. Microalbuminuria in patients with NIDDM: an overview. Diabetes Care. 1996;19:79-89.

Bojestig M, Arnqvist HJ, Hermansson G, Karlberg BE, Ludvigsson J. Declining incidence of nephropathy in insulin-dependent diabetes mellitus. N Engl J Med. 1994;330:15-18.

Brennan DR. CAPD in IDDM: initial treatment strategies. Diabetes Spectrum. 1994;7:327-328.

Coonrod BA, Ellis D, Becker DJ, et al. Predictors of microalbuminuria in individuals with IDDM. Pittsburgh Epidemiology of Diabetes Complications Study. Diabetes Care. 1993;16:1376-1383.

DeFronzo RA. Diabetic nephropathy: etiologic and therapeutic considerations. Diabetes Reviews. 1995;3:510-548.

DeFronzo RA. Diabetic nephropathy. In: Therapy for Diabetes Mellitus and Related Disorders. 3rd ed. Alexandria, Va: American Diabetes Association; 1998:338-363.

Irvin B. Maximizing nutrition therapy at every stage of diabetic nephropathy. Diabetes Spectrum. 1997;10:304-308.

Ismail N, Becker B, Strzelczyk P, Ritz E. Renal disease and hypertension in non-insulin-dependent diabetes mellitus. Kidney Int. 1999;55:1-28.

Kelly M. Chronic renal failure. Am J Nurs. 1996;96(1):36-37.

Kleinbeck C. Challenges of diabetes and dialysis. Diabetes Spectrum. 1997; 10:135-141.

Kopple JD. Nutrition management of non-dialyzed patients with chronic renal failure. In: Nutrition Management of Renal Disease. Kopple JD, Shaul GM, eds. Baltimore: Williams and Wilkins; 1997:479-531.

Mogensen CE, Vestbo E, Poulsen PL, et al. Microalbuminuria and potential confounders. A review and some observations on variability of urinary albumin excretion. Diabetes Care. 1995;18:572-579.

Smulders YM, Rakic M, Stehouwer CDA, Weijers RNM, Slaats EH, Silberbusch J. Determinants of progression of microalbuminuria in patients with NIDDM. Diabetes Care. 1997;20:999-1005.

Striker G. Report on a workshop to develop management recommendations for the prevention of progression in chronic renal disease. J Am S Neph. 1995;5:1537-1540.

Wang S-L, Head J, Stevens L, Fuller JH. WHO Multinational Study Group. Excess mortality and its relation to hypertension and proteinuria in diabetic patients. Diabetes Care. 1996;19:305-312.

Learning Assessment: Post-Test Questions

Nephropathy   8

1 Which of the following statements is most accurate about diabetic nephropathy?
   A Both persons with type 1 and type 2 diabetes can expect to experience some symptoms and complications of nephropathy
   B Persons with microalbuminuria and proteinuria usually have some retinopathy
   C Persons with diabetes experience the same frequency of kidney dysfunction as individuals who do not have diabetes
   D Symptoms of nephropathy usually occur 2 to 3 years after diagnosis is first made

2 The functions of the kidney include
   A The removal of water, urea, iron, and protein from the body
   B The maintenance of blood volume and formation of 1,25 dehydroxy vitamin D
   C The conservation of potassium and excretion of sodium
   D The inhibition of erythropoietin production

3 Structural changes characteristic of nephropathy include
   A Basement membrane thickening which precedes mesangial expansion
   B The presence of microalbuminuria, indicating that the nephrons have closed
   C Hypertrophy of the nephrons, which usually occurs in the second decade after diagnosis
   D Elevated blood pressure in 70% of individuals at the time of diagnosis

4 Which of the following is not true?
   A Diabetes accounts for more than 35% of new cases of ESRD
   B In persons with diabetes over age 45, the incidence of ESRD has increased 12-fold
   C The incidence of ESRD in Hispanics and Native Americans is 6 times higher than Caucasians with diabetes
   D The development of ESRD in African Americans with diabetes is approximately equal to that occurring in Caucasians with diabetes

5 The stage of renal disease at which microalbuminuria first appears is:
   A Functional changes
   B Structural change
   C Incipient nephropathy
   D Overt nephropathy

6 At which stage of kidney involvement has improved glycemic control been shown to restore alterations in function?
   A Functional changes
   B Structural changes
   C End stage renal disease
   D Overt nephropathy

7 What effect does declining renal function have on insulin catabolism?
   A Increased insulin catabolism prolongs insulin availability resulting in hypoglycemia
   B Increased insulin catabolism decreases availability of insulin resulting in hyperglycemia
   C Decreased insulin catabolism prolongs insulin availability resulting in hypoglycemia
   D Decreased insulin catabolism decreases insulin availability resulting in hyperglycemia

8 Risk factors for diabetic nephropathy include all of the following except:
   A Hypertension
   B Hyperglycemia
   C Low-protein diet
   D Genetic predisposition

9 SW is having a creatinine clearance test. You explain to her that this is a test that involves:

A The collection of all urine for 24 hours

B A urine specimen treated with dye and its clearance timed

C A blood specimen used to measure her creatinine

D Urine collected for a 4-hour period

10 Which strategy would be best to consider when evaluating treatment options for ESRD?

A Begin to plan treatment when serum creatinine reaches 1.8 mg/dL

B Discuss only the treatment option the healthcare team believes is best for the person

C Suggest patient meet others who are experiencing the treatment modalities being considered

D Recommend that patients with cardiovascular disease not consider renal transplantation

11 GA is a 75-year-old man who has had diabetes for 25 years. He has glaucoma, is blind in the left eye, and has limited mobility. He has requested no renal replacement for his ESRD. In your discussion with him, which of the following would you not include?

A No renal replacement for ESRD is an option but it will result in death

B This decision must be made when he is in a nonuremic state

C His wife, children, and grandchildren should be his reason to live and choose treatments that keep him alive

D Resources are available to him and his family if he decides on no renal replacement

12 Which of the following are not manifestations of renal failure in diabetes?

A Weight gain, pedal edema, shortness of breath

B Hiccups, nausea, vomiting

C Skeletal fractures, changes in concentration, muscle cramping

D Diaphoresis, shaking, blurred vision

13 JC is being taught about prevention of renal damage. Important information for her to know would be:

A Kidney infections should be treated with aminoglycoside drugs

B Contrast dyes can be used for diagnostic tests if necessary

C If she has symptoms of a urinary tract infection, she should push fluids and call her provider after 2 to 3 days if symptoms persist

D She should empty her bladder after sexual intercourse

14 The laboratory test indicating first evidence of kidney damage is:

A Serum creatine levels over 2 mg/dL on 2 occasions

B Blood urea nitrogen over 20 mg/dL on more than 1 occasion

C Protein excretion = 3.6 g/24 hours

D Albumin excretion rate of 30 to 300 mg/day on 3 different occasions

15 A limitation of renal transplant surgery as a treatment option for nephropathy is:

A The new kidney will function effectively for a limited time only

B The patient must use immunosuppressive drugs for the remainder of his/her life

C Patient will still need to follow a restricted diet to avoid damaging the new kidney

D Blood glucose levels are not likely to change or will improve only slightly following surgery

16 An effective approach for the diabetes educator in dealing with the psychosocial issues associated with end-stage renal disease is:

A Reassure the patient it is not his or her fault

B Assess on an on-going basis the patient's ability to cope with loss and handle complex treatments

C Use scare tactics only when other attempts to get patient's attention fail

D Recommend support groups only when the patient seems motivated to succeed

See next page for answer key.

Post-Test Answer Key

Nephropathy   8

1	B		9	A
2	B		10	C
3	A		11	C
4	D		12	D
5	C		13	D
6	A		14	D
7	C		15	B
8	C		16	B

A Core Curriculum for Diabetes Education
Diabetes and Complications

Diabetic Neuropathy

Martha Mitchell Funnell, MS, RN, CDE
Michigan Diabetes Research and Training Center
University of Michigan Medical Center
Ann Arbor, Michigan

Eva L. Feldman, MD, PhD
Department of Neurology
University of Michigan Medical School
Ann Arbor, Michigan

Introduction

1 Diabetes is the most common cause of peripheral neuropathy in the Western world and is responsible for significant patient morbidity.[1] A person with diabetes has a 15% chance in his or her lifetime to develop a neuropathic foot ulcer that requires an amputation. The cost to society is large.[2,3] In the United States, the national annual direct cost of diabetic foot ulcers is estimated to be $5 billion with an indirect cost rate of $400 million.[2] The average Medicare expenditure between 1995 and 1996 for a diabetic patient was $15 309 compared to $5 226 for Medicare patients in general and 25% of these dollars went to the treatment of foot ulcers.[2] Thus, diabetic neuropathy is a common complication, causing significant morbidity and financial burden.

2 Diabetic neuropathy is thought to be the result of insulin deficiency.[4] It encompasses a group of clinical and subclinical syndromes with varying etiologies and manifestations. Each syndrome is characterized by either diffuse or focal damage to the peripheral somatic or autonomic nerve fibers.[5] Treatment is directed toward prevention, early diagnosis, optimal glucose control, relief of symptoms, avoidance of secondary complications, and patient education for self-care.[6]

3 Patients with neuropathy are often told that the pain and other symptoms of neuropathy are just something they will have to live with. Because diabetic neuropathy has become the subject of intense research interest, however, there is new understanding of its causes and breakthroughs in treatment. The purpose of this chapter is to review the pathogenesis and approaches to the prevention and management of diabetic polyneuropathy as it affects the peripheral nervous system and identify areas of current and future research.

Objectives

Upon completion of this chapter, the learner will be able to
1 Define diabetic neuropathy.
2 Explain the role of blood glucose control in the development and treatment of peripheral neuropathies.
3 List pharmacological and nonpharmacological treatments for peripheral neuropathy.
4 List the clinical manifestations of diffuse sensory neuropathy.
5 List the classifications and clinical manifestations of autonomic neuropathy.
6 State the primary symptom for each of the focal neuropathies.
7 Describe the key information about neuropathy that should be taught to all patients with diabetes.

Key Definitions

1 *Apoptosis.* A form of cellular suicide or programmed death that occurs in a cell when confronted with toxic or metabolic insults.

2 *Axon.* The central core of nerve fiber that conducts impulses away from the nerve cell body.

3 *Myelin.* The fat-like substance forming a sheath around certain nerve fibers.

4 *Neuron.* The structural and functional unit of the nervous system.

5 *Plexus.* A network made up of nerve fibers.

6 *Radiculopathy.* Disease condition of the nerve roots in spinal nerves.

7 *Sorbitol.* A crystalline alcohol that is the intermediate product in the metabolism of glucose in the nerve and other tissues.

Definition of Diabetic Neuropathy

1 *Diabetic neuropathy* is a descriptive term for a clinical or subclinical disorder that occurs in people with diabetes.[1] Although it is often thought of in terms of the more common symptoms of pain and numbness, diabetic neuropathy is actually a large group of sensory and autonomic syndromes with a wide range of manifestations.[1,5]

2 *Diabetic neuropathy* is defined as peripheral nerve dysfunction that occurs in people with diabetes, is of a type known to be more prevalent among people with diabetes, and cannot be attributed to any other disease.[1,5]

3 The diagnosis and staging of diabetic neuropathy are based on signs, symptoms, and objective measures. Objective evidence (eg, electrodiagnostic and sensory tests) is needed to detect subclinical neuropathy. *Clinical neuropathy* is diagnosed and defined through symptoms, clinical signs, and objective measures, and it is subdivided into syndromes according to the distribution of peripheral nervous system involvement. The 2 subcategories of clinical neuropathy are *diffuse polyneuropathy* (multiple nerve involvement), which includes both sensory and autonomic impairment, and *focal neuropathy* (individual nerve involvement)[1] (see Table 9.1).

4 Each syndrome has a characteristic clinical presentation and course, although multiple syndromes may overlap and coexist.[1,5] The majority of patients experience diffuse neuropathies consisting of distal symmetric, primarily sensory, polyneuropathies that are often accompanied by diabetic autonomic neuropathy.

5 The diffuse neuropathies are generally chronic, frequently progressive, and associated with increased morbidity and mortality.[5] The focal neuropathies occur less often, are generally acute in onset, and are often self-limited.

Occurrence of Diabetic Neuropathy

1 Reliable prevalence estimates of diabetic neuropathy have been difficult to obtain because of the lack of standard diagnostic measures and consensus in diagnostic criteria.[7] Diabetic neuropathy occurs with similar frequency in patients with type 1 or type 2 diabetes and also in patients with various forms of acquired diabetes.[8,9]

Table 9.1. Classification and Staging of Diabetic Neuropathy

Class I: Subclinical Neuropathy*
1 Abnormal electrodiagnostic tests (EDX)
   A Decreased nerve conduction velocity
   B Decreased amplitude of evoked muscle or nerve action potential
2 Abnormal quantitative sensory testing (QST)
   A Vibratory/tactile
   B Thermal warming/cooling
   C Other
3 Abnormal autonomic function tests (AFT)
   A Diminished sinus arrhythmia (beat-to-beat heart rate variation)
   B Diminished sudomotor function
   C Increased pupillary latency

Class II: Clinical Neuropathy
1 Diffuse neuropathy
   A Distal symmetric sensorimotor polyneuropathy
   • Primarily small-fiber neuropathy
   • Primarily large-fiber neuropathy
   • Mixed
   B Autonomic neuropathy
   • Genitourinary autonomic neuropathy
      — Bladder dysfunction
      — Sexual dysfunction
   • Gastrointestinal autonomic neuropathy
      — Gastric atony
      — Diabetic enteropathy
   • Cardiovascular autonomic neuropathy
   • Hypoglycemic unawareness
   • Sudomotor dysfunction
   • Abnormal pupillary function
2 Focal neuropathy
   A Mononeuropathy
   B Mononeuropathy multiplex
   C Plexopathy
   D Radiculopathy
   E Cranial neuropathy

* Neurological function tests are abnormal but no neurological symptoms or clinically detectable neurological deficits indicative of a diffuse or focal neuropathy are present. Class I, subclinical neuropathy, is further subdivided into class IA if an AFT or QST abnormality is present, class IB if EDX or AFT and QST abnormalities are present, and class IC if an EDX and either AFT or QST abnormalities or both are present.

Source: Adapted with permission from Greene et al.[1]

2 Estimates for the prevalence of neuropathy generally average 50% and are dependent on the duration and extent of diabetes. Pirat's classic study[10] reported 8% prevalence at the time of diagnosis (mostly in older type 2 patients) that increased in a linear manner to 50% after 25 years. Similar results are reported from several studies of both type 1 and type 2 patients. In the United Kingdom, the prevalence of neuropathy reached 44% in elderly patients with diabetes.[11] In an Italian study, a simple neuropathy screening instrument that evaluates vibration, light touch, and ankle reflexes was administered to 8757 patients with diabetes and 32% had clinical findings diagnostic of neuropathy.[12] In the Rochester Diabetic Neuropathy study, which is now ongoing for 15 years, 54% of persons with type 1 and 45% of persons with type 2 diabetes have neuropathy.[13]

3 Sensory symptoms (eg, pain) are reported by an average of 20% of people with diabetes in the United States.[1] As many as 20% to 30% of patients with long-standing diabetes have symptoms of gastroparesis.[1] Carpal tunnel syndrome occurs in 4% to 29% of people with both types of diabetes and also is related to duration.[14]

4 In type 1 diabetes, the prevalence of neuropathy parallels the duration and severity of hyperglycemia.[15] While this prevalence is probably also true in type 2 diabetes, undiagnosed patients may present initially with symptoms and signs of sensory and/or autonomic neuropathy and subsequently be diagnosed with diabetes.[5] The most likely explanation for this occurrence is the insidious nature of type 2 diabetes, which may be present but undiagnosed for years.

5 Diabetic neuropathy can be considered an extremely common problem that ultimately affects about half of all patients with diabetes.[1]

Pathology

1 The *nervous system* is divided into the central nervous system and the peripheral nervous system. The *peripheral nervous system* is made up of the autonomic nervous system (sympathetic and parasympathetic) and the sensorimotor nervous system. Autonomic nerves control involuntary functions, sensory nerves send information from the skin and internal organs about how things feel, and motor nerves send commands from the brain to the body about movement.

2 Most of the pathology of diabetic neuropathy occurs in the peripheral nervous system, although there may be some central nervous system involvement. All types of neuropathies occur in the peripheral nervous system.[8]

3 Diabetic neuropathy is believed to be a disease involving acute nerve fiber abnormalities, followed by more chronic nerve fiber injury, atrophy, and loss. The loss of nerve fibers is gradual and progressive. The most common pathological lesion is axonal loss with secondary loss of myelin.[4]

4 Neuropathies occur secondary to axonal degeneration that progresses from the distal to the proximal portions of the neurons. The distal portions are eventually more seriously affected. This process is further affected by microvascular dysfunction and blunted nerve fiber regeneration and is linked with the effects of hyperglycemia on the cell constituents of peripheral nerve tissue and its supporting connective tissue and vascular elements.[4]

Pathogenesis

1 The association between diabetes and neuropathic symptoms in the legs and feet was first made by John Rollo over 200 years ago,[16] yet the pathogenesis of diabetic neuropathy is still unknown.[17] The Diabetes Control and Complications Trial (DCCT) confirmed the long-held idea that hyperglycemia is the cause of neuropathy.[15] Cigarette smoking is also implicated as a risk factor for neuropathy.[1]

2 Results from the DCCT provided evidence that intensive therapy decreased the risk for neuropathy by 60% in a large sample of participants with type 1 diabetes and slows the development and progression of abnormal autonomic tests.[15] There is less direct evidence of the influence of glucose control on the risk for neuropathy for patients with type 2 diabetes.[18-20] Poor glucose control, hypoinsulinemia, age, race, obesity, and duration of diabetes all have been linked with diabetic peripheral neuropathy in people with type 2 diabetes.[20] Overall, diabetic neuropathy is thought to result from the interaction between multiple metabolic, genetic, and environmental factors.[21,22] Prevention efforts are focused primarily on improved glucose control throughout the course of all types of diabetes.[23]

3 There are several theories about why neuropathy occurs: accumulation of polyols in the nerve cells leading to cofactor depletion, nerve glycosylation, and nerve hypoxia. Underlying these seemingly divergent ideas is the fact that each of these changes in nerve metabolism leads to cellular oxidative stress.[24] Thus, the idea is emerging that there is one unifying ultimate insult that damages nerves.[4]

A One theory is based on the conversion of glucose to sorbitol by the enzyme aldose reductase and secondary depletion of NADPH, a required cofactor for cellular oxidative defense.

- Unlike most other cells, nerve cells do not need insulin to move glucose into the cell. Therefore, high levels of blood glucose lead to high levels of glucose within the nerve cells.
- Once inside the cell, glucose is reduced to sorbitol by an enzyme called aldose reductase (sorbitol pathway). Sorbitol is then oxidized to fructose by the enzyme sorbitol dehydrogenase (polyol pathway). These reactions deplete the cell of needed cofactors in the NADPH/NADP family.
- In diabetes, peripheral nerve glucose, sorbitol, and fructose levels are elevated, which alters normal intracellular metabolism and depletes the nerve of the NADP family of cofactors required to detoxify superoxide.[4] Accumulation of superoxides (ie, cellular oxidative stress) is toxic to nerves. Specific aldose reductase inhibitors have been shown to improve nerve function by preventing the conversion of glucose to sorbitol and the depletion of needed NADP family cofactors.[25]

B Additional theories are related to glycosylation of nerve myelin and microvascular disease. It has been hypothesized that glycosylation of cellular proteins, which is similar to the processes resulting in glycosylation of nerve myelin, leads to loss of function of enzymes needed for antioxidative defense.[25]

C The theory of hypoxia is based on the decreased blood flow and oxygen tension found in people with diabetes. Decreased perfusion to peripheral nerve tissue leads to accumulation of free oxygen radicals, which further promotes oxidative stress.[25] Large blood vessel occlusive disease alone does not produce peripheral neuropathy.[4]

D In summary, the common link for the theories on nerve damage is *oxidative stress*. Hyperglycemia produces a series of interrelated changes in the way cofactors, proteins, and lipids are metabolized. These changes generate molecules called free oxygen radicals. Because free oxygen radicals are toxic to cells, they cause oxidative stress. Oxidative stress robs cells of oxygen and growth factors. This result is death of the nerve cells also known as *apoptosis*.[25]

4 The pathology of autonomic neuropathy is related to axonal degeneration and fiber loss in the sympathetic and parasympathetic systems. The nerves of the gastrointestinal systems also are affected.[26] A metabolic basis for autonomic abnormalities similar to sensory polyneuropathy has been suggested, although autoimmunity also may play a role.[5,27]

5 The cause of focal neuropathies is thought to be acute ischemic events (probably microthrombi and platelet thrombi).

Diagnosis

1 Diagnosis is a process that involves excluding other potential causes of the signs and symptoms presented by the patient. Reported symptoms generally are of limited use in making a diagnosis of sensory neuropathy.[13] However, monofilament testing for decreased tactile perception[28,29] and clinical signs such as loss of ankle reflexes and decreased vibration sensation can be used as screening measures for sensory neuropathy.[30] Objective measures such as electrodiagnostic testing along with a standardized neurological exam are used to confirm and stage the diagnosis.[12,30]

2 Physical assessment of the person with diabetes needs to include evaluation of temperature, position sense, muscle strength, and deep tendon reflexes.[30]

A Pain and light-touch sensations can be assessed using vibration and monofilament testing.

B Temperature sensation can be assessed by touching a cool piece of metal (eg, a tuning fork, metal end of a reflex hammer) to the skin and asking the patient to describe the temperature.

C Position sense is assessed by flexing and extending the big toes and asking that the patient describe the position.

D Vibration sensation is assessed by applying a 128-Hz tuning fork to the distal first metatarsal head.

E Routine assessment of blood pressures (lying, sitting, standing), cardiac status, and symptoms of autonomic neuropathic syndromes also need to be performed. There are now systems to diagnose autonomic neuropathy that include lying-to-standing pulse variability and rhythmic breathing (eg, Anscore by Boston Medical). The Valsalva-stimulated R-R response is sensitive to changes in autonomic function.[31]

3 Annual risk categorization using monofilament testing for early detection of insensitive feet can have a substantial impact on focusing patient education to prevent injury, sepsis, ulceration, and amputation.[28,29,32,33]

Treatment

1 Treatment generally is palliative; supportive; and aimed at symptom relief, optimizing blood glucose control, addressing psychosocial distress or depression, protecting the feet, and providing patient self-management education.[6]

2 Both pharmacological and nonpharmacological therapies may be useful for pain relief. Improved control of blood glucose levels may result in a decrease in symptoms for some patients. However, pain may initially worsen as a result of nerve regeneration.

3 Aldose reductase inhibitors (ARIs), alpha-lipoic acid, nerve growth factors and antioxidants are also being studied as potential therapies for neuropathy.

Overview of Diffuse Sensory Neuropathies

1 *Distal symmetric sensorimotor polyneuropathy* (sensory neuropathy) primarily involves the sensory nerves. It is the most widely known form of neuropathy, and affects approximately three fourths of patients with neuropathy.[1] Sensory deficits and symptoms begin in the distal portions of the lower extremities and progress to the upper extremities, in a "stocking-glove" pattern. Lower extremities tend to be affected more seriously than upper extremities. The nerve fiber loss and atrophy is progressive. The spread of symptoms is related to increasing duration and severity of this syndrome.[34] Manifestations in the early stages can include deterioration of nerve function and development of subtle sensory-motor deficits with minimal or absent symptoms. In the late stage, bands of sensory loss in the trunk area may occur.[1,34]

2 Sensory neuropathy can be viewed as a disease of progressive nerve fiber loss, atrophy, and injury. The signs and symptoms depend on the class and stage of nerve fiber loss (Table 9.2). Small fiber involvement impairs pain and temperature sensations, large fiber involvement produces diminished proprioception and light-touch sensation, and motor nerve damage results in loss of muscle tone. Most patients experience damage to more than one type of nerve.[1,34]

Diffuse Sensory Neuropathies

1 The following are characteristics of subclinical sensory neuropathy.
   A The early stages of sensory neuropathy may be manifested as deterioration of nerve function and development of subtle sensory-motor deficits. Most patients have minimal symptoms at this stage.
   B Some patients may present with neurological deficits that are found during a physical examination or with complications, such as undetected trauma to an insensate foot.[35]
   C Nerve fiber damage may be so mild that it is not apparent even with a careful physical examination but is evident only with nerve function testing or nerve biopsy.[34,36,37]

Table 9.2. Sensory Neuropathy Deficits and Symptoms

Syndrome	Symptoms
Small-fiber damage	• Loss of ability to detect temperature • Pins-and-needles, tingling, or burning sensations • Pain, usually worse at night • Numbness or loss of feeling • Cold extremities • Swelling of feet • Pain on contact with clothing or bedsheets
Large-fiber damage	• Abnormal or unusual sensations • Loss of balance • Unable to sense position of toes and feet • Unable to feel feet when walking
Motor nerve damage	• Loss of muscle tone in hands and feet
Foot deformities	• Callus formation • Charcot joint • Misshapen or deformed toes and feet • Open sores or ulcers on feet

2 The following are characteristics of small-fiber neuropathy.

A Several types of spontaneous pain or discomfort may be associated with small-fiber neuropathy. Patients most often experience paresthesias (spontaneous uncomfortable sensations), dysesthesias (contact paresthesias), or pain. The pain is described as superficial and burning, shooting or stabbing, or bone-deep and aching or tearing and is generally more severe at night. The pain can become disabling in and of itself. Depression may occur as a result of unremitting pain, sleep disturbance, or diminished quality of life.[38,39] In contrast, some patients have subjective symptoms of numbness or cold feet. Undetected trauma, particularly on the feet, is common.[40]

B Sensory loss appears to correspond closely with the degree of nerve damage. However, pain corresponds more closely with independent processes such as fiber regeneration or structural deformities.[41]

C In acute painful neuropathy, the pain develops and then remits in less than 6 months. Precipitous weight loss may occur. In chronic painful neuropathy, symptoms appear and stabilize for more than 6 months or disappear and are replaced by dense sensory deficits such as numb or cold feet.[42]

D Diminished deep tendon reflexes of the Achilles tendon and diminished temperature, pinprick, and monofilament sensations may be early signs of neuropathies.[43] Sensory impairment is clinically significant because it can predispose to ulceration.[44]

E Symptoms may occur in the absence of neurological deficits on physical examination.[34]

3 The following are characteristics of large-fiber neuropathy.

   A Impaired balance and diminished proprioception and joint position sense are symptoms of large-fiber damage. Pain is usually absent, and sensory ataxia may occur in the most severe cases.[34]

   B Clinical signs may include absent or reduced vibration sensation, impaired touch or pressure sensation, and diminished ankle reflexes.[5,34]

   C Foot deformities are primarily the result of damage to the large-fiber nerves in association with small-fiber distal motor and autonomic abnormalities.[44-46] (See Chapter 4, Diabetic Foot Care and Education, in Diabetes and Complications, for more information.)

4 The following are characteristics of motor neuropathy.

   A Causes muscle weakness and atrophy of intrinsic foot muscles, leaving the pull of the long muscles unopposed.

   B Ankle weakness and foot drop can then result.[5]

Treatment of Diffuse Sensory Neuropathies

1 Treatment is focused on glycemic control, pain management, relief from the depression that often accompanies chronic pain, and protecting deformed feet.[6]

2 Improved glycemic control may decrease the pain and other symptoms for some patients, although the pain may initially worsen.[6]

3 Nonpharmacological therapies include walking to ease leg pains, gentle massage, stretching exercises, avoiding alcohol, relaxation exercises, biofeedback, hypnosis, acupuncture,[47] use of percutaneous[48] or transcutaneous[49] nerve stimulation units, body stockings or pantyhose to keep clothes away from hypersensitive skin, brief cold water foot soaks, and referral to a pain control clinic.

4 Pharmacological therapy usually begins with the use of nonnarcotic analgesics such as ibuprofen and sulindac. Other agents are added as needed: amitriptyline (Elavil), nortriptyline or doxepin; and gabapentin (Neurontin) or carbamazepine (Tegretol).[50-52] Tramadol (Alcar) has been shown to be effective for pain relief.[53]

5 Lamb's wool padding, gentle filing of calloused areas, and specially made shoes, molded insoles or other orthotic devices can be used to protect deformed areas of the feet. Referral to a podiatrist or orthotic specialist is needed to identify abnormal weight-bearing and to prescribe mechanical measures to compensate.[54]

Complications of Diffuse Sensory Neuropathies

1 Neuropathic syndromes can culminate in sensory and motor denervation that parallel severity and proximal extension of the sensory loss. These tertiary complications include insensitivity to pain, limb deformity, ulceration, neuroarthropathy, infection, and amputation.[5,34]

2 Neuropathic foot ulcers often occur in areas where the fat pad is decreased and callus form as a result of weight-bearing pressure. Autonomic neuropathy further leads to decreased perspiration and a tendency for dry, cracked skin and infection. Injuries may remain unnoticed due to diminished sensation until infection develops.[44-46]

3 Neuropathic arthropathy (Charcot joint) can occur when motor function remains intact but sensation is impaired. The small joints of the foot (tarsals, metatarsals) are most commonly affected. The foot is swollen, red, and painless in the early stages. Multiple fractures, fragmentations, and disarticulations occur in the later stages. As the patient continues to walk on the injured, insensate foot, marked deformities occur such as a flattened arch and "bag of bones" appearance.[55,56]

4 Treatment for these complications is aimed at removing continued trauma, appropriate footwear, patient education concerning foot-care practices and aggressive follow-up and surveillance.[6,40,54]

Overview of Autonomic Neuropathies

1 Diabetic autonomic neuropathies (DAN) can occur with all types of diabetes and can affect any system in the body.[27]

A The relationship of DAN to sensorimotor polyneuropathy varies, but these conditions generally coexist.

B As many as 50% of patients with peripheral neuropathy may also have DAN.[27]

2 Because morbidity and mortality rates are closely linked to DAN, early diagnosis and treatment is of critical importance.[27,31]

3 The most common classifications of DAN, accompanying clinical manifestations, and interventions and self-management education for each syndrome are shown in Table 9.3.

Autonomic Neuropathies

1 The following are characteristics of genitourinary impairment.[27,31]

A Both bladder and sexual functioning may be affected.

B Bladder dysfunction generally occurs in association with distal symmetric polyneuropathy. It is also associated with impotence among males.

• Afferent autonomic fibers transmit bladder fullness sensations (normally with 300 cc urine) and efferent parasympathetic fibers promote bladder contraction during micturition. Efferent sympathetic nerves maintain sphincter tone. Damage can occur to all of these nerves; however, motor function usually remains intact.

• Symptoms of a neurogenic bladder are usually insidious and progressive. In the early stages, the sensation of the need to void may be blunted. This infrequent urination may be misinterpreted as decreased polyuria due to improved blood glucose control. In later stages, difficulty in emptying the bladder, dribbling, and overflow incontinence may occur.

Table 9.3. Diabetic Autonomic Neuropathies

Classification	Symptoms and Signs	Intervention/Patient Education
Genitourinary Neurogenic bladder	• Diminished urinary frequency • Incomplete or difficult bladder emptying • Frequent urinary tract infections • Bladder residual volume >150 mL	• Schedule urination every 2 hours • Prevention, signs, and symptoms of UTIs; seek treatment immediately • Credé maneuver, palpation for bladder distention, self-catheterization
Sexual dysfunction	*In males* • Retrograde ejaculation • Impotence *In females* • Diminished vaginal lubrication • Decreased frequency of orgasm	• Report symptoms to healthcare team; therapeutic options, uses, and potential side effects • Referral to impotence clinic, urologist/gynecologist
Gastrointestinal Gastroparesis	• Early satiety • Postprandial fullness • Postprandial hypoglycemia	Therapeutic options, uses, and potential side effects; appropriate meal planning and frequent meals; importance of blood glucose control; frequent blood glucose monitoring; insulin adjustment; referral to a gastroenterologist
Intestinal	• Nocturnal diarrhea • Fecal incontinence	Adequate fiber and fluid intake and physical activity to prevent constipation; therapeutic options, uses, and potential side effects; importance of blood glucose control; judicious use of laxatives; bowel program, relaxation, or biofeedback
Cardiovascular Orthostatic hypotension	• Postural hypotension	Safety measures to prevent falls; rise slowly from a recumbent position; proper use of elastic body stockings; importance of blood glucose control; therapeutic options, uses, and potential side effects
Cardiac denervation	• Fixed heart rate • Painless MI, sudden death	• Avoid heavy exercise and straining • Prevent hypoglycemia
Abnormal cardiovascular response to exercise	• Hypotension with exercise	• Avoid aerobic exercise
Impaired insulin counterregulation	• Unawareness of hypoglycemia • "Brittle" diabetes	Frequent blood glucose monitoring, particularly before driving; prevention of hypoglycemia; wearing appropriate identification; treatment of hypoglycemia, including glucagon; appropriate blood glucose goals
Sudomotor	• Areas of symmetrical anhidrosis • Gustatory sweating	• Check for fissures and lubricate feet daily; prevent heatstroke through avoidance of high heat and humidity • Avoid offending foods
Pupillary	• Decreased/absent responsiveness to light • Decreased pupil size	Caution regarding night driving; use of nightlights; safety measures to avoid falls such as turning on lights when entering a dark room

- Bladder insensitivity is diagnosed by a cystometrogram. A postvoid urine residual volume of greater than 150 mL by ultrasound or postvoid catheterization confirms bladder dysfunction.
- Untreated neurogenic bladder often leads to urinary tract infections as a result of urinary stasis. These frequent infections may accelerate deterioration of renal function. More than 2 urinary tract infections per year among men and 3 among women are indicative of the need for further evaluation of bladder function.
- Treatment involves frequent palpation for bladder fullness, scheduled urination every 2 to 4 hours during waking hours using manual suprapubic pressure (Credé method) to ensure that the bladder is empty, vigorous antibiotic therapy for infections, and parasympathomimetic drug treatment (eg, bethanechol) to improve nerve contraction. Self-catheterization may be needed if the nerves to the bladder are severely damaged.
- Stress the need for frequent, complete urination; the signs and symptoms of urinary tract infections; and the importance of early treatment for infections. Patients can also be taught to palpate for bladder fullness.

C Sexual dysfunction is common among people with diabetes. As many as 75% of men and 35% of women experience sexual problems due to diabetic neuropathy.[5]

D Male sexual dysfunction involves impotence and retrograde ejaculation.[57]

- Retrograde ejaculation is unusual and results in damage to the efferent sympathetic nerves that normally coordinate the simultaneous closure of the internal vesicle sphincter and relaxation of the external vesicle sphincter. Symptoms include cloudy urine following intercourse and decreased volume of ejaculate. Retrograde ejaculation is diagnosed by the presence of oligospermia, azoospermia, and abnormal amounts of sperm in postcoital urine. Retrograde ejaculation may respond to the use of an antihistamine, desipramine, or phenylephrine.[57] Fertility may be possible by instructing patients to have intercourse with a full bladder or by harvesting sperm from the urine and artificially inseminating them into the prospective mother.
- Impotence is marked by impairment or loss of erectile ability sufficient for intercourse despite a normal libido.[40] Organic impotence is gradual in onset (from partial to complete in 2 years), is partner nonspecific, and characterized by lack of erections during sleep.[57]
- Diagnosis of impotence involves ruling out other causes such as medications (eg, alcohol, antihypertensives), hormonal deficiencies, or psychological causes. The assessment process can include penile blood flow and pressure measurements, blood hormone levels, nocturnal tumescence (eg, Snap Gauge®) testing, and referral to a urologist for further evaluation. Diabetic autonomic neuropathy is specifically associated with diminished or absent testicular pain sensation to pressure and loss of perineal sensation. The sensations are lost because of parallel loss of somatic and autonomic sacral segments.[5,27,57]
- Offer the patient and his partner referral to an impotence clinic or urologist for diagnosis and counseling. Review therapeutic options and their costs and benefits. Treatment options include suction devices that produce an erection, rigid or semirigid penile prostheses (surgical implants), prostaglandin urethral suppositories (Muse®), injection of prostaglandins (Captoject®) directly into the corpus cavernosum to produce erection, or oral medications (sildenafil citrate [Viagra™]).

- Management for impotence often begins with use of an oral medication and progresses to other options as needed.

E Female sexual dysfunction involves difficulties in arousal, decreased vaginal lubrication during stimulation, and anorgasmia despite a normal libido.[5,27,57]

- Symptoms such as dyspareunia, decreased lubrication, and delayed or absent orgasmic response need further assessment.
- Management includes application of estrogen or lubricant vaginal creams and referral to a gynecologist. Offer the patient and her partner referral for counseling.

F Sexual difficulties not related to autonomic neuropathy include loss of libido related to depression as a result of diabetes and its complications and the frequent occurrence of yeast and other vaginal infections in women with diabetes.

G It is important for diabetes educators to address sexual concerns because these issues may be difficult for patients to discuss. Discuss sexual function, the potential for diabetes-related problems, and the need to bring problems to the attention of providers. Offer to include patients' partners in the discussion and point out the importance of their inclusion in treatment decisions.

2 The following are characteristics of gastrointestinal impairment.

A Virtually all of the gastrointestinal system has autonomic innervation.[26] The parasympathetic nervous system stimulates intestinal and gastric peristalsis, dopaminergic innervation inhibits gastric peristalsis, and the sympathetic nervous system inhibits gastric emptying.

B In persons without diabetic autonomic neuropathy, liquids empty from the stomach in about 30 minutes and solid foods in about 150 minutes. If the nerves are affected by autonomic neuropathy, gastric emptying of both liquids and solids may be delayed. Most of the evidence supports vagal nerve dysfunction as responsible for motility disturbances. Upper gastrointestinal dysfunction may involve the esophagus, stomach, and upper small intestine.

- Symptoms of gastroparesis (delayed gastric emptying) can include heartburn, reflux, anorexia, early satiety, nausea, abdominal bloating, erratic blood glucose levels due to delayed absorption of food, and vomiting undigested food eaten several hours or days earlier.[26] Signs associated with gastroparesis include weight loss and gastrospasm, although delayed gastric emptying can also occur without symptoms.[26]
- Visualization of the upper gastrointestinal tract with a barium series is useful to rule out obstruction and determine liquid-phase gastric emptying. A solid-phase gastric emptying phase study is the most specific way to diagnose delayed gastric emptying.[26]
- Treatment includes referral to a dietitian for a low-fat/low-fiber diet; multiple small and mostly liquid meals eaten throughout the day. Referral to a gastroenterologist, medications to decrease inhibition of gastric motility such as metoclopramide (Reglan) or octreotide taken 30 minutes before all meals and snacks and at bedtime, or other medications that increase the motility of the stomach such as erythromycin or bethanechol may be useful. In the most severe stages jejunostomy tube feedings may be necessary.
- Although normalizing blood glucose levels may improve gastric emptying, the presence of gastroparesis complicates balancing insulin doses with food absorption.

Frequent monitoring of preprandial and postprandial blood glucose levels is needed to detect hypoglycemia and hyperglycemia and determine the insulin dose. Rapid-acting insulin (lispro) is probably not appropriate for some patients with gastroparesis, although some find it useful if taken after the meal.

C Lower intestinal tract dysfunction is the result of damage to the efferent autonomic nerves. This damage leads to hypotonia and poor contraction of the smooth muscles to the gut, which results in constipation.

- Constipation is fairly common and has been reported in up to 60% of all patients with diabetes. Treatment involves increasing fiber in the diet while avoiding excess fiber; judicious use of laxatives; adequate hydration; increased activity; stool softeners and bulk laxatives such as psyllium (Metamucil); and medications such as metoclopramide (Reglan) or neostigmine (Prostigmin) to increase intestinal mobility.[26]

- Decreased small intestinal motility may lead to an overgrowth of the normal intestinal bacteria and diarrhea. Diarrhea can also occur as a result of hypermotility without bacterial overgrowth.[26]

- Although constipation is more common, diarrhea is usually more troublesome to patients. Diarrhea may be nocturnal, intermittent with constipation, and associated with fecal incontinence; it may occur without cramping or pain. Treatment involves the use of antibiotics (eg, tetracycline) to decrease the bacterial overgrowth (if confirmed by a hydrogen breath test). Medications that may be useful for slowing intestinal motility are loperamide, codeine, diphenoxylate hydrochloride, or atropine sulfate. Fiber and psyllium may increase stool bulk and consistency. In addition, some patients may benefit from biofeedback, relaxation, and bowel training. Early treatment of diarrhea may help prevent the development of incontinence.[26]

- A discussion of these symptoms as they relate to diabetes is an important part of patient education. Stress the need to inform providers of symptoms to allow for early detection and treatment. Explanations of diagnostic tests, test results, and therapies are also needed.

3 The following are characteristics of cardiovascular impairment.

A Cardiovascular dysfunction is associated with abnormalities in heart rate control and vascular dynamics. Parasympathetic nerves slow the heart rate, and sympathetic nerves increase the speed and force of heart contractions and stimulate the vascular tree to increase the blood pressure. Cardiovascular impairment is present in up to 40% of patients with diabetes. The three major associated syndromes are orthostatic (postural) hypotension, cardiac denervation syndrome, and abnormal cardiovascular response to exercise.[5,31]

B Blood pressure is normally maintained upon standing by a sympathetic reflex that increases the heart rate and by peripheral vascular resistance in association with an increase in norepinephrine levels. *Orthostatic (postural) hypotension* is defined as a drop in systolic blood pressure of more than 30 mm Hg or a diastolic drop of more than 10 mm Hg within 2 minutes of changing from a supine to standing position. This syndrome occurs late in diabetes and signals advanced autonomic impairment.

- Orthostatic hypotension, which results from blood pooling in the feet, can occur without symptoms but often is accompanied by dizziness, light-headedness, weakness, visual impairment, or syncope.[5,31] This places the patient at risk for injury from falls and also may lead to edema.

- Assessment of blood pressure and pulse rates in the lying, sitting, and standing positions is needed for all patients who have diabetes. Greater accuracy in the assessment can be achieved by having the patient rest in a supine position, then stand quietly while the blood pressure is measured at 1-minute intervals for 3 to 5 minutes.[5,31]
- Treatment of symptoms involves raising the head of the bed 30 degrees at night, standing in stages, increasing venous pressure with supportive elastic body stockings that are applied while supine, and wearing an antigravity suit. Other treatments include correcting hypovolemia through glycemic control, increased salt intake, and/or fludrocortisone to expand the plasma volume.[5,31]
- Pharmacologic therapies can include fludrocortisone, yohimbine, metoclopramide, phenylephrine (Neo-Synephrine® nasal spray), ephedrine, midodrine (ProAmatine®), beta blockers, clonidine, and somatostatin analog.[5,31]
- Patient education is focused on proper application and use of elastic body stockings and instructing patients to rise slowly from a recumbent position.

C Cardiac denervation syndrome is defined as a fixed heart rate that does not change in response to stress, exercise, breathing patterns, or sleep. This syndrome results from both parasympathetic and sympathetic system impairment. Initially, parasympathetic tone decreases, which causes a relative increase in sympathetic tone and an increase in heart rate. Progressive impairment of sympathetic tone causes a gradual slowing of the heart. Over time, both parasympathetic and sympathetic tone become impaired.[5,31]

- Initially, a fixed heart rate of 100 to 120 beats per minute is common. In the later stages, the fixed heart rate will be in the range of 80 to 100 beats per minute. The heart rate is unresponsive to stress, exercise, or tilting.[5,31]
- In the later stages, patients may suffer myocardial ischemia or myocardial infarction without experiencing pain. The resulting delay or failure to seek treatment contributes to increasing mortality rates. These patients are also at risk for cardiac arrhythmias and sudden death.[5,31]
- Cardiac denervation is assessed using specific devices designed to test for autonomic neuropathy (eg, Anscore by Boston Medical) or an EKG to check the pulse or heart rate during deep breathing (6 breaths per minute) or before or after a Valsalva maneuver or exercise. No variation in heart rate is indicative of cardiac nerve damage.[5,31] Teach patients with this syndrome to avoid heavy exercise, aerobic exercise, and straining. Stress testing is needed before initiating any type of exercise program. In addition, these patients need to be carefully evaluated prior to initiation of intensive insulin therapy because of the risk of hypoglycemia, which can result in cardiac arrhythmias.[5,31]

D Some people with diabetic autonomic neuropathy may lose their normal increased cardiac output and vascular tone response to exercise and become hypotensive with aerobic activity.[5,31]

4 The following are characteristics of impaired insulin counterregulation.

A Maintaining blood glucose levels during times of food deprivation and increased insulin action depends on glucagon secretion and the adrenergic nervous system.[5,27] The acute counterregulatory response to low blood glucose levels is an increase in the secretion of glucagon, epinephrine, growth hormone, cortical, and glucose production by the liver. Patients with autonomic neuropathy may have a defective adrenergic nervous system and defective glucagon secretion, both of which lead to impaired counterregulation and recovery from hypoglycemia. The decline in glucagon and epinephrine responses greatly diminishes the counterregulatory response and increases the risk for severe hypoglycemia.[5,27]

- In people with type 1 diabetes, the normal glucagon response begins to deteriorate within 5 years of diagnosis. The epinephrine response declines with increasing duration of type 1 diabetes and may be lost after 15 to 30 years. Absent glucagon and epinephrine responses greatly increase the risk for severe hypoglycemia. The counterregulatory mechanism in type 2 diabetes is largely unknown.[5,27]

B People with diabetes of long duration may further experience hypoglycemia unawareness due to a lack of the classic adrenergic warning signs of hypoglycemia: anxiety, nervousness, sweating, and palpitations. These patients may instead develop neuroglycopenia when hypoglycemic and become lethargic, irritable, dull, confused, and lose consciousness or have a seizure.[5,27] Frequent hypoglycemia also increases the risk for hypoglycemia unawareness.

- Assess hypoglycemia warning symptoms and episodes of severe hypoglycemia and coma during patient visits.
- The costs and benefits of more liberal glucose goals need to be discussed with patients who have hypoglycemia unawareness. Although improved metabolic control may reverse autonomic neuropathy, normoglycemia poses considerable risk for these patients. Long-acting insulins with only small premeal boluses are generally recommended. These patients may benefit from using rapid-acting insulin (lispro) based on carbohydrate intake given just before or after a meal by injection or from insulin pump therapy.[5,27]
- Patient education includes prevention of hypoglycemia, appropriate treatment, the value of frequent home blood glucose monitoring, caution while driving, and wearing appropriate diabetes identification. Teach family members the signs and treatment of hypoglycemia, including glucagon administration. Blood glucose awareness training may improve functional capacity.[5,27,58]

5 The following are characteristics of sudomotor dysfunction.

A This type of autonomic neuropathy is commonly manifested by anhidrosis in a stocking-glove pattern with compensatory hyperhidrosis of the face and trunk. Bilateral symmetrical loss of the thermoregulatory response and gustatory sweating in response to foods (cheese, spicy foods) that normally induce salivation may also occur.[27]

B Patients rarely think to report abnormal sweating. However, this symptom is important because of the potential for heat stroke and foot ulcers. A careful history should be taken and the feet should be examined for dryness and fissures at each visit.[5,27]

C Propantheline hydrobromide or scopolamine patches may help to relieve severe gustatory sweating.[5,27]

D Patient education includes inspection for fissures and lubrication for dry feet; avoidance of hot, spicy or other offending foods; and prevention of hyperthermia and heat stroke.

6 The following are characteristics of an abnormal pupillary response.

A The iris is innervated by both parasympathetic and sympathetic nerve fibers.

Sympathetic nerve fibers cause the pupils to dilate and are generally more severely affected. Abnormal pupillary responses are related to duration of diabetes.[5,27,59]

B Slow dilation of pupils in response to darkness may be observed during clinical examination. Patients may report slow adaptation when entering a dark room.

C Stress using caution during night driving, the importance of turning on lights when entering a dark room, and using nightlights in darkened hallways and bathrooms to help prevent injuries.

Overview of Focal Neuropathies

1 The various focal neuropathies occur acutely and unpredictably. They are not specific to diabetes and are not thought to be related to duration of diabetes. There are no strategies to prevent these neuropathies or provide early detection, but this is offset by their self-limiting nature.[5,14,35]

2 The primary symptom of the focal neuropathies is acute local pain. Abnormal nerve conduction that corresponds to the distribution of a single nerve, multiple peripheral nerves, the brachial or lumbosacral plexus, or nerve roots will be noted. Focal neuropathies often occur in middle-aged patients or those with sensorimotor polyneuropathy. There are 4 major focal neuropathies.[5,14,35]

Focal Neuropathies

1 The following are characteristics of mononeuropathy and mononeuropathy complex.

A Isolated neuropathies of one or several nerves are more common among people with diabetes. *Carpal tunnel syndrome* (compression or entrapment of the median nerve of the wrist) is the most common and occurs 3 times more often in people with diabetes than in the general population.[5,14,35] Other common mononeuropathies include the ulnar nerve of the elbow leading to weakness and loss of sensation over the palmer aspect of the fourth and fifth fingers, the radial nerve of the upper arm leading to wrist drop, the lateral cutaneous nerve in the thigh, and the peroneal nerve at the head of the fibula leading to foot drop.

B Diagnosis is based on pain, wrist or foot drop, and abnormal electrodiagnostic studies.

C Treatment usually consists of surgical release of the nerve, physical therapy, or protection from further trauma using wrist splints, elbow pads, and ankle braces.

2 The following are characteristics of *plexopathy* (femoral neuropathy).

A The sacral plexus and femoral nerves are generally affected, causing a pain that extends from the hip to the anterior and lateral surface of the thigh. Pain is generally worse at night and can cause weakness and wasting of thigh flexion and knee extension muscles. Femoral neuropathy occurs most often among older adults.[5,14,35]

B Nonnarcotic or simple analgesics may be used to relieve pain, which generally remits spontaneously but may recur periodically. Some groups advocate immunosuppression as a form of therapy although there are no controlled trials to substantiate its use.[60]

3 The following are characteristics of *radiculopathy* (intercostal neuropathy).

A This focal neuropathy occurs as a result of damage to the nerve root. It is singular and unilateral with pain localized to the chest or abdominal wall. The patient generally presents with absent cutaneous sensation and pain or dysesthesia that is worse at night. Profound weight loss may also occur.

B Nonnarcotic or simple analgesics may help control the pain, which generally remits spontaneously in 6 to 24 months.[61]

4 The following are characteristics of *cranial neuropathy* (diabetic ophthalmoplegial).

A The third cranial nerve is most often affected. The onset is generally abrupt with headache, eye pain, or dysesthesias of the upper lip that precede palsy by several days. Ptosis is marked, and the affected person is unable to move the eye, although the pupil is generally spared. Cranial neuropathy occurs most often in older adults.[59]

B Use of an eye patch for the affected eye may be helpful. Pain and oculomotor function will gradually improve after several weeks, with full recovery in 3 to 5 months.[59]

Key Educational Considerations

1 The importance of foot inspection and care must be emphasized for patients with peripheral neuropathy (see Chapter 4, Diabetic Foot Care and Education, in Diabetes and Complications, for detailed information).

2 Periodically assess patients with diabetes for the presence of modifiable risk factors for peripheral neuropathy, including hyperglycemia, alcohol abuse, smoking, and hypertension.

A Refer patients to counseling or organizations such as Alcoholics Anonymous if an alcohol abuse problem is identified.

B Discuss the added risks of smoking, and ascertain the patient's thoughts about stopping. Provide information about local smoking cessation programs. Some patients may find that medications such as Wellbutrin® and Zyban™ (bupropion) can both lower or raise blood glucose levels). Nicotine patches, inhalers, or gum will help in their attempts to stop smoking.

3 Because some manifestations of neuropathy (eg, sexual dysfunction, incontinence) may be embarrassing for the patient to discuss, tactfully assess these problems during each visit.

4 Inform patients about the symptoms of neuropathy and encourage them to report these symptoms to their provider. The topic of neuropathy, pain management, and treatment options can provide the basis for an effective group discussion because the symptoms commonly occur.

5 Because this content can be difficult to teach and learn, avoid detailed explanations of the complexity of the nervous system. Instead, present a simplified explanation such as "Some nerves send information about how things feel, others tell the body to move, and others control automatic body functions." Focus teaching on what patients need to know (eg, symptoms and treatment) and discuss pathology only as needed. Visual aids can enhance understanding.

A Reinforce the relationship between hyperglycemia and neuropathic pain. If patients are interested, discuss specific options for improving blood glucose levels.

B Open-ended questions will often yield information about the use of alternative therapies for pain.

C Offer patients options for both nonpharmacological and pharmacological treatment for pain.

D Because most therapies to relieve neuropathic pain take time to work, prepare patients for the delay and encourage them to give the therapies a fair trial.

E The depression that can accompany painful neuropathy may act as a barrier to learning and treatment. Therefore, treatment for depression is needed in conjunction with treatment for neuropathy. Focus teaching on what the patient can do to ease the discomfort and prevent other related problems. Include significant others in education and offer options for support.

F Encourage patients with neuropathy to stay informed about new research studies and findings about the treatment of neuropathy.

G Provide education about complications with sensitivity and only after the patient's readiness to hear this information has been determined. Point out the value of early detection and the hope for future treatment of neuropathy.

Self-Review Questions

1 Define diabetic neuropathy.

2 List the classifications of peripheral neuropathy and the respective subcategories.

3 List therapies that are available for sensory neuropathies.

4 Describe the major symptoms, clinical manifestations, and treatments for the autonomic neuropathies.

5 Describe what patients with diabetes need to know about neuropathy.

Learning Assessment: Case Study 1

WJ is a 56-year-old African-American male with a 10-year history of type 2 diabetes, which has been treated with glyburide 5.0 mg bid for the last 7 years. His HbA1c was 9.4% when measured today. He does not monitor his blood glucose levels at home because his insurance does not cover the cost of strips. He reports some blurred vision but denies any other symptoms of hyperglycemia. WJ is 5 ft 8 in (173 cm) tall and weighs 198 lb (90 kg). He was told by his doctor to follow a 1600-calorie ADA diet but states that he is hungry all of the time when he tries this diet; it also doesn't include the food that he likes to eat, particularly ethnic foods. His weight has been stable at about 200 lb (91 kg) since diagnosis. He is married, has 3 grown children, and works as a carpenter. WJ is a deacon in his church and describes church and family as important to him.

He presents today with burning and tingling sensations in his feet and occasional dizziness on standing. When asked about his greatest concern about his diabetes, he tells you it is that he has "lost his nature" for the past 3 months. His wife calls you aside and tells you that she is concerned because he appears to be depressed and is withdrawing from friends and family. She is also concerned because recently his cigarette smoking has increased to 2 packs per day. He reports some alcohol intake on social occasions.

On physical examination, WJ has diminished bilateral vibratory and monofilament responses, and dry feet. His sitting blood pressure is 148/84 mm Hg, supine is 136/82, and standing is 100/76. His fasting blood glucose is 196 mg/dL. When asked, he tells you he takes care of his feet by soaking them in vinegar once per week.

Questions for Discussion

1 What information does WJ need to address his educational concerns?

2 What strategies can you use to address his psychosocial concerns?

Discussion

1 Provide information about the potential costs and benefits of improved glycemic control. If he is interested, offer WJ options for achieving better blood glucose control through an individualized meal plan, addition of another oral agent, or initiation of insulin therapy.

2 Offer WJ a referral for a new meal plan that better fits his lifestyle and preferred/cultural eating patterns and facilities safe initiation of insulin therapy. Because his wife does the shopping and cooking for the family, ask if he would like for her to attend this appointment.

3 Offer to provide self-management education about the following.
  A Neuropathy
  B Foot care, emphasizing lubrication, appropriate footwear, and daily inspection; point out that soaking and use of vinegar may cause dryness
  C Home blood glucose monitoring, including resources for strips
  D Safety issues related to carpentry work, particularly protecting feet and legs

4 Determine whether WJ understands the impact of smoking on complications and his health in general. If he is interested, provide information about methods and support that are available for smoking cessation.

5 Assess WJ's interest in medication to treat his impotence. Offer to include his wife in this discussion.

6 Offer referral to a social worker or counselor for evaluation and nonpharmacological treatment of depression and/or to a physician for pharmacological treatment of depression. Ask if his minister could be helpful with this issue and offer referral to a diabetes support group.

Learning Assessment: Case Study 2

SH is as 36-year-old female who has had type 1 diabetes for 22 years. When she comes to the clinic, you notice that she has several fading bruises and is wearing a cervical collar. She tells you that she was recently in an automobile accident while on her way to pick up her children at school. She states that she had no warning signals of hypoglycemia and has no memory of the accident. Witnesses said that SH was driving erratically prior to the accident and was very confused when the ambulance arrived. Her blood glucose was 26 mg/dL in the emergency room, so she assumes that a low blood glucose level caused her collision.

Her husband is with her for this visit and is very concerned for her safety and that of their children because she frequently drives them to school and various activities. He is also concerned because her diabetes was not recognized initially by the paramedics who did not notice her medical identification bracelet. He tells you that he has had to tell her on several occasions that her blood glucose is low based on her behavior, but she had not noticed any symptoms. The most recent episode occurred last night, shortly after dinner. SH usually treats her hypoglycemia with a regular soft drink, but has noticed that her blood glucose level does not always respond as quickly as in the past.

While reviewing SH's blood glucose records you notice fairly wide variations in her glucose levels. She attributes these variations to the stress of her new part-time job. She denies nausea and vomiting but tells you that sometimes she has to force herself to eat all of the food in her meal plan because she feels full.

Questions for Discussion

1 What information does SH need related to her safety?

2 What additional information is needed to better assess the potential causes of SH's hypoglycemia?

Discussion

1 Provide information to SH and her husband about hypoglycemia unawareness, treatments other than beverages (glucose gel or tubes of cake icing), glucagon administration, training in recognition of subtle symptoms, and the need for frequent blood glucose monitoring.

2 Discuss steps with SH that she can take to protect herself and others when driving, including testing her blood glucose prior to driving to be sure that it is over 100 mg/dL, testing frequently during extended driving times, carrying a form of treatment at all times, and having more visible diabetes identification.

3 Address SH's concerns and those of her husband about her safety when he is not available. Determine her comfort with providing coworkers and children with information about the signs of hypoglycemia and actions to take if they notice these signs.

4 Assess the cause of SH's erratic blood glucose levels through more comprehensive record-keeping that includes the times and amounts of food eaten, timing, types and doses of insulin, and activity and stress levels. Review these records after 2 to 3 weeks, and consider gastric emptying studies if the erratic glucose levels do not appear to be related to these other factors.

Acknowledgments

This work was supported in part by the Juvenile Diabetes Research Foundation, Center for the Study of the Complications in Diabetes, and the National Institutes of Diabetes and Digestive and Kidney Diseases of the National Institutes of Health (grant number NIH5P60-DK20572)

References

1 Greene DA, Feldman EL, Stevens MJ, Sima AAF, Albers JW, Pfeifer MA. Diabetic neuropathy. In: Porte D Jr and Sherwin R, eds. Diabetes Mellitus. East Norwalk, Ct: Appleton & Lange; 1997:1009-1076.

2 Bloomgarden ZT. American Diabetes Association annual meeting, 1999: nephropathy and neuropathy. Diabetes Care. 2000;23:549-556.

3 Resnick HE, Valsania P, Phillips CL. Diabetes mellitus and nontraumatic lower extremity amputation in black and white Americans: the National Health and Nutrition Examination Survey Epidemiologic Follow-up Study, 1971-1992. Arch Intern Med. 1999;159:2470-2475.

4 Stevens MJ, Feldman EL, Thomas T, Greene DA. Pathogenesis of diabetic neuropathy. In: Veves A, ed. Clinical Management of Diabetic Neuropathy. Totowa, New Jersey: Humana Press. 1998:13-48.

5 Windebank AJ, Feldman EL. Diabetes and the nervous system. In: Aminoff MJ, ed. Neurology and General Medicine. Churchill Livingstone. 2001:341-364.

6 Feldman EL, Stevens MJ, Greene DA. Clinical management of diabetic neuropathy. In: Veves A, ed. Clinical Management of Diabetic Neuropathy. Totowa, New Jersey: Humana Press; 1998:89-105.

7 Vinik AI, Park TS, Stansberry KB, Pittenger GL. Diabetic neuropathies [In Process Citation]. Diabetologia. 2000;43:957-973.

8 Feldman EL, Stevens MJ, Russell JW, Greene DA. Diabetic neuropathy. In: Taylor S, ed. Current Review of Diabetes. Current Medicine; 1999:71-83.

9 Feldman EL, Stevens MJ, Greene DA. Diabetic neuropathy. In: Turtle JR, Kaneko T, Osato S, eds. Diabetes in the New Millennium. Sydney: The Endocrinology and Diabetes Research Foundation of the University of Sydney. 1999:387-401.

10 Pirart J. Diabetes mellitus and its degenerative complications; a prospective study of 4,400 patients observed between 1947 and 1973. Diabetes Care. 1978;1:168-188.

11 Young MJ, Boulton AJM, Macleod AF, Williams DRR, Sonksen PH. A multicentre study of the prevalence of diabetic peripheral neuropathy in the United Kingdom hospital clinic population. Diabetologia. 1993;36:150-154.

12 Fedele D, Comi G, Coscelli C, et al, and Italian Diabetic Neuropathy Committee. A multicenter study on the prevalence of diabetic neuropathy in Italy. Diabetes Care. 1997;20:836-843.

13 Dyck PJ, Kratz KM, Karnes JL, et al. The prevalence by staged severity of various types of diabetic neuropathy, retinopathy, and nephropathy in a population-based cohort: The Rochester Diabetic Neuropathy Study. Neurology. 1993;43:817-824.

14 Freimer M, Brushart TM, Cornblath DR, Kissel JT. Entrapment neuropathies. In: Mendell JR, Kissel JT, Cornblath DR, eds. Diagnosis and Management of Peripheral Nerve Disorders. New York: Oxford University Press; 2001:592-638.

15 The Diabetes Control and Complications Trial Research Group. The effect of intensive treatment of diabetes on the development and progression of long-term complications in insulin-dependent diabetes mellitus. N Engl J Med. 1993;329:977-986.

16 Rollo J. Cases of Diabetes Mellitus. London: C. Dilly; 1798.

17 Greene DA, Stevens MJ, Feldman EL. Diabetic neuropathy: scope of the syndrome. Am J Med. 1999;107(2B):2S-8S.

18 Turner RC. The UK Prospective Diabetes Study (UKPDS): a review. Diabetes Care. 1998;21(suppl 3):535-538.

19 Azad N, Emanuele NV, Abraira C, et al. The effects of intensive glycemic control on neuropathy in the VA cooperative study on type II diabetes mellitus (VA CSDM). J Diabetes Complications. 1999;13:307-313.

20 Gaster B, Hirsch IB. The effects of improved glycemic control on complications in type 2 diabetes. Arch Intern Med. 1998;158:134-140.

21 Molyneaux LM, Constantino MI, McGill M, Zilkens R, Yue DK. Better glycemic control and risk reduction of diabetic complications in Type 2 diabetes: comparison with the DCCT. Diabetes Res Clin Pract. 1998;42:77-83.

22 Klein R, Klein BE, Moss SE. Relation of glycemic control to diabetic microvascular complications in diabetes mellitus. Ann Intern Med. 1996;124:90-96.

23 Greene DA, Stevens MJ, Feldman EL. Glycemic control. In: Dyck PJ, Thomas PK, eds. Diabetic Neuropathy. Philadelphia: W.B. Saunders; 1998:297-315.

24 Feldman EL, Russell JW, Sullivan KA, Golovoy D. New insights into the pathogenesis of diabetic neuropathy. Curr Opin Neurol. 1999;12:553-563.

25 Greene DA, Obrosova I, Stevens MJ, Feldman EL. Pathways of glucose-mediated oxidative stress in diabetic neuropathy. In: Packer L, Rosen P, Tritschler HJ, King GL, Azzi A, eds. Antioxidants in Diabetes Management. New York: Marcel Dekker; 2000:111-119.

26 Malagelada J-R. Gastrointestinal disorders. In: Veves A, ed. Clinical Management of Diabetic Neuropathy. Totowa, New Jersey: Humana Press; 1998:243-256.

27 Freeman R. Diabetic autonomic neuropathy: an overview. In: Veves A, ed. Clinical Management of Diabetic Neuropathy. Totowa, New Jersey: Humana Press. 1998:181-208.

28 Sosenko JM, Sparling YH, Hu D, Welty T, Howard BV, Lee E, Robbins DC. Use of the Semmes-Weinstein monofilament in the Strong Heart Study. Risk factors for clinical neuropathy. Diabetes Care. 1999;22:1715-1721.

29 Valk GD, de Sonnaville JJ, van Houtum WH, et al. The assessment of diabetic polyneuropathy in daily clinical practice: reproducibility and validity of Semmes Weinstein monofilaments examination and clinical neurological examination. Muscle Nerve. 1997;20:116-118.

30 Feldman EL, Stevens MJ, Thomas PK, Brown MB, Canal N, Greene DA. A practical two-step quantitative clinical and electrophysiological assessment for the diagnosis and staging of diabetic neuropathy. Diabetes Care. 1996;17:1281-1289.

31 Deliargyris EN, Nesto RW. Autonomic neuropathy and heart disease. In: Veves A, ed. Clinical Management of Diabetic Neuropathy. Totowa, New Jersey: Humana Press. 1998:209-226.

32 Kumar S, Fernando DJ, Veves A, Knowles EA, Young MJ, Boulton AJ. Semmes-Weinstein monofilaments: a simple, effective and inexpensive screening device for identifying diabetic patients at risk of foot ulceration. Diabetes Res Clin Pract. 1991;13:63-67.

33 Mueller MJ. Identifying patients with diabetes mellitus who are at risk for lower-extremity complications: use of Semmes-Weinstein monofilaments. Phys Ther. 1996;76:68-71.

34 Zochodne DW. Diabetic neuropathies: features and mechanisms. Brain Pathol. 1999; 9:369-391.

35 Mendell JR. Diabetic neuropathies. In: Mendell JR, Kissel JT, Cornblath DR, eds. Diagnosis and Management of Peripheral Nerve Disorders. New York: Oxford University Press; 2001:373-399.

36 Meh D, Denislic M. Subclinical neuropathy in type I diabetic children. Electroencephalogr Clin Neurophysiol. 1998; 109:274-280.

37 American Diabetes Association Report and Recommendations of the San Antonio Conference on Diabetic Neuropathy. Neurology. 1988;37:1000-1004.

38 Galer BS, Gianas A, Jensen MP. Painful diabetic polyneuropathy: epidemiology, pain description, and quality of life. Diabetes Res Clin Pract. 2000;47:123-128.

39 Benbow SJ, Cossins L, MacFarlane IA. Painful diabetic neuropathy. Diabet Med. 1999;16:632-644.

40 Smieja M, Hunt DL, Edelman D, Etchells E, Cornuz J, Simel DL. Clinical examination for the detection of protective sensation in the feet of diabetic patients. International Cooperative Group for Clinical Examination Research. J Gen Intern Med. 1999;14:418-424.

41 Belgrade MJ. Following the clues to neuropathic pain. Distribution and other leads reveal the cause and the treatment approach. Postgrad Med. 1999;106:127-140.

42 Boulton AJM, Scarpello JHB, Armstrong WD, Ward JD. The natural history of painful diabetic neuropathy—a 4-year study. Postgrad Med J, 1983;59:556-559.

43 Thomas PK. Classification, differential diagnosis, and staging of diabetic peripheral neuropathy. Diabetes. 1997;46(suppl 2): S54-S57.

44 Boyko EJ, Ahroni JH, Stense V, Forsberg RC, Davignon DR, Smith DG. A prospective study of risk factors for diabetic foot ulcer. The Seattle Diabetic Foot Study. Diabetes Care. 1999;22:1036-1042.

45 de Sonnaville JJ, Colly LP, Wijkel D, Heine RJ. The prevalence and determinants of foot ulceration in type II diabetic patients in a primary health care setting. Diabetes Res Clin Pract. 1997;35:149-156.

46 Sauseng S, Kastenbauer T, Sokol G, Irsigler K. Estimation of risk for plantar foot ulceration in diabetic patients with neuropathy. Diabetes Nutr Metab. 1999;12:189-193.

47 Abuaisha BB, Costanzi JB, Boulton AJ. Acupuncture for the treatment of chronic painful peripheral neuropathy. Diabetes Research and Clinical Practice. 1998; 39:115-121.

48 Hazma MA, White PF, Craig WF, et al. Percutaneous electrical nerve stimulation: a novel analgesic therapy for diabetic neuropathic pain. Diabetes Care. 2000;23:365-370.

49 Kumar D, Alvaro MS, Julka IS, Marshall HJ. Diabetic peripheral neuropathy. Effectiveness of electrotherapy and amitriptyline for symptomatic relief. Diabetes Care. 1998;21:1322-1325.

50 Joss JD. Tricyclic antidepressant use in diabetic neuropathy. Ann Pharmacother. 1999;33:996-1000.

51 Backonja MM. Gabapentin monotherapy for the symptomatic treatment of painful neuropathy: a multicenter, double-blind, placebo-controlled trial in patients with diabetes mellitus. Epilepsia. 1999; 40(suppl 6):S57-S59.

52 Morello CM, Leckband SG, Stoner CP, Moorhouse DF, Sahagian GA. Randomized double-blind study comparing the efficacy of gabapentin with amitriptyline on diabetic peripheral neuropathy pain [see comments]. Arch Intern Med. 1999;159:1931-1937.

53 Harati Y, Gooch C, Swenson M, et al. Maintenance of the long-term effectiveness of tramadol in treatment of the pain of diabetic neuropathy. Diabetes and its Complications. 2000;14:65-70.

54 Giurini JM, Rosenblum BI, Lyons TE. Management of the diabetic foot. In: Veves A, ed. Clinical Management of Diabetic Neuropathy. Totowa, New Jersey: Humana Press. 1998:303-318.

55 Wilson M. Charcot foot osteoarthropathy in diabetes mellitus. Mil Med. 1991; 156:563-569.

56 Edmonds ME, Watkins PJ. Plantar neuropathic ulcer and Charcot joints: risk factors, presentation, and management. In: Dyck PJ, Thomas PK, eds. Diabetic Neuropathy. Philadelphia: W.B. Saunders Company. 1998:398-406.

57 Webster L. Diabetic impotence: pathogenesis and treatment. In: Veves A, ed. Clinical Management of Diabetic Neuropathy. Totowa, New Jersey: Humana Press; 1998:227-242.

58 Cox DJ, Gonder-Frederick L, Julian DM, Clark, W. Long-term follow up evaluation of blood glucose awareness training. Diabetes Care. 1994;17:1-5.

59 Asbury AK, Aldredge H, Hershberg R, Fisher CM. Oculomotor palsy in diabetes mellitus: A clinicopathological study. Brain. 1970;93:555-566.

60 Jaradeh SS, Prieto TE, Lobeck LJ. Progressive polyradiculoneuropathy in diabetes: correlation of variables and clinical outcome after immunotherapy. J Neurol Neurosurg Psychiatry. 1999; 67:607-612.

61 Longstreth GF. Diabetic thoracic polyradiculopathy: ten patients with abdominal pain. Am J Gastroenterol. 1997;92:502-505.

Suggested Readings

American Diabetes Association. Diabetic neuropathy (consensus statement). Diabetes Care. 1996;19(suppl 1):S67-S71.

Barnett JL. Will the nausea ever end? Diabetes Forecast. 1997;50(7):31-35.

Bernstein G. Gastroparesis: dealing with a sluggish stomach. Diabetes Self-Management. 1997;14(2):62-65.

Boulton AJ. Guidelines for diagnosis and outpatient management of diabetic peripheral neuropathy. European Association for the Study of Diabetes, Neurodiab. Diabetes and Metabolism. 1998;24(suppl 3):55-65.

Clark WL. When diabetes strikes a nerve. Countdown. 2000;21(2):38-42.

Cowley EP, Haines ST. Return to a regular life. Diabetes Forecast. 1996; 49(12):42-48.

Culverwell M. Possible answer for some men with diabetes. Countdown. 2000;21(2): 43-46.

Dejgaard A. Pathophysiology and treatment of diabetic neuropathy. Diabetic Medicine. 1998;15:97-112.

Donaghue KC. Autonomic neuropathy: Diagnosis and impact on health in adolescents with diabetes. Hormone Research. 1998;50(suppl 1):33-37.

Dyck J, Davies JL, Wilson DM, Service FJ, Melton LJ III, O'Brien PC. Risk factors for the severity of diabetic polyneuropathy. Diabetes Care. 1999;22:1479-1486.

Eastman RC, Garfield SA. Prevention and treatment of microvascular and neuropathic complications of diabetes. Primary Care. 1999;26:791-807.

Haines ST. Treating constipation in the patient with diabetes. Diabetes Educ. 1995;21:223-232.

Haire-Joshu D, Glasgow R. Smoking and diabetes (technical review). Diabetes Care. 1999; 22:1887-1898.

Herman WA, Greene DA. Microvascular complications of diabetes. In: Haire-Joshu D, ed. Management of Diabetes Mellitus. Perspectives of Care Across the Life Span. 2nd ed. St. Louis: CV Mosby, 1996:234-80.

Lyrenas EB, Olsson EHK, Arvidsson UC, Orn TJ, Spjuth JH. Prevalence and determinants of solid and liquid gastric emptying in unstable type I diabetes. Diabetes Care. 1997;20:413-418.

Maser RE. Autonomic neuropathy: patient care. From research to practice. Diabetes Spectrum. 1998;11:224-256.

Merio R, Festa A, Bergmann H, et al. Slow gastric emptying in type I diabetes: relation to autonomic and peripheral neuropathy, blood glucose, and glycemic control. Diabetes Care. 1997;20:419-423.

Pendergast JJ. Diabetic autonomic neuropathy. Practical Diabetology. 2001;20(1):7-15.

Poirier—Solomon L. Celebrating your sexuality. Diabetes Forecast. 2001;54(5):39-41.

Sands ML, Shetterly SM, Franklin GM, Hamman RF. Incidence of distal symmetric (sensory) neuropathy in NIDDM. Diabetes Care. 1997;20:322-329.

Tanenberg RJ, Pfeifer MA. Neuropathy: The "forgotten" complication. Diabetes Forecast. 2000;53(12):56-61.

Vinik AI. Diagnosis and management of diabetic neuropathy. Clinics in Geriatric Medicine. 1999;15:293-320.

Waldman SD. Diabetic neuropathy: diagnosis and treatment for the pain management specialist. Current Review of Pain. 2000;4:383-387.

Yeap BB, Russo A, Faser RJ, Wittert GA, Horowitz M. Hyperglycemia affects cardiovascular autonomic nerve function in normal subjects. Diabetes Care. 1996;19:880-882.

Zangaro GA, Hull MM. Diabetic neuropathy: pathophysiology and prevention of food ulcers. Clinical Nurse Specialist. 1999;13:57-68.

Learning Assessment: Post-Test Questions

Diabetic Neuropathy

9

1 Diabetic neuropathy is described as a condition:
   A Which affects the peripheral and central nervous systems almost equally
   B With a narrowly defined range of manifestations
   C Which results from the interaction of multiple metabolic, genetic, environmental factors
   D That is not generally painful but is self-limiting in nature

2 The most common pathological lesion in diabetic neuropathy is:
   A Excitation of postsynaptic membranes
   B Demyelinization and atrophy of peripheral nerve axons
   C Loss of active transport mechanisms of neurotransmitters
   D Loss of white matter within the central nervous system

3 The prevalence of subclinical signs and clinical symptoms of neuropathy in diabetes appear to be strongly correlated with:
   A The degree of pain and numbness experienced by patient
   B Number of episodes of symptomatic hypoglycemia
   C Duration of the disease
   D Type of medication used to achieve glycemic control

4 A characteristic that distinguishes the focal neuropathies from the diffuse polyneuropathies is
   A Focal neuropathies are associated with higher rates of morbidity and mortality
   B Diffuse polyneuropathies are asymmetrical
   C Focal neuropathies are acute in onset and self-limiting in nature
   D Diffuse polyneuropathies are limited to autonomic impairment only

5 Teach patients with peripheral neuropathy that improved glycemic control may:
   A Improve long-term effects but cause increased discomfort temporarily
   B Have no long-term effect but temporarily increase discomfort
   C Improve long-term prognosis and result in rapid relief of symptoms
   D Have no long-term effect but result in rapid relief of symptoms

6 The most common mononeuropathy is involvement of the:
   A Median nerve, leading to carpal tunnel syndrome
   B Peroneal nerve, leading to foot drop
   C Radial nerve, leading to wrist drop
   D Ulnar nerve, leading to weakness and paresthesia of the lateral fingers

7 Treatment for orthostatic hypotension related to diabetic autonomic neuropathy with cardiovascular involvement includes all of the following except:
   A Increased salt intake
   B Use of supportive elastic body stockings
   C Improved glycemic control
   D Raise head of bed to a 60-degree angle

8 MH is a 45-year-old female who has had type 1 diabetes for 25 years. She takes her insulin regularly but does not do SMBG. Concerned about several recent episodes of hypoglycemia, her provider recently reevaluated her medication and self-care and found them to be adequate. Lab tests were unremarkable. What would be the most likely cause of her hypoglycemia?
   A Autoimmune response to the insulin
   B Development of gastroparesis with delayed gastric emptying
   C Inappropriate glucagon response
   D Changes in renal clearance of insulin

9 Diabetic neuropathy includes all of the following except:
A Acute nerve fiber abnormalities
B Chronic nerve fiber injury or loss
C Atrophy of longer peripheral nerve axons
D Central nervous system impairment due to macrovascular dysfunction

10 LM is a 55-year-old female with type 2 diabetes who was recently diagnosed with a neurogenic bladder. Which of the following interventions would be most helpful to her at this stage:
A Teach her the Credé method
B Encourage an aerobic exercise program to promote circulation
C Instruct her on the signs and symptoms of urinary tract infections
D Teach her self-catheterization

11 LM is least likely to experience dysfunction or disruption of:
A Efferent autonomic fibers signaling bladder fullness
B Efferent sympathetic fibers responsible for maintaining sphincter tone
C Efferent parasympathetic fibers promoting bladder contraction
D Motor function signaling release of urine

12 JH complains of altered sensations and impaired feeling. Which test would you expect to be ordered to determine nerve conduction velocity?
A Electrodiagnostic test (EDX)
B Quantitative sensory testing (QST)
C Autonomic function test (AFT)
D Transcutaneous nerve stimulation (TENS)

13 The most accurate statement about gastroparesis associated with autonomic neuropathy and gastrointestinal dysfunction is that:
A Involvement is limited to the stomach
B It is easily detected because of occurrence of overt signs and symptoms
C It is treated with a high-protein/high-fiber diet to stimulate motility
D It requires frequent monitoring of preprandial and postprandial blood glucose levels.

See next page for answer key.

Post-Test Answer Key

Diabetic Neuropathy

9

1	C		**8**	B
2	B		**9**	D
3	C		**10**	A
4	C		**11**	D
5	A		**12**	A
6	A		**13**	D
7	D			

A Core Curriculum for Diabetes Education
Diabetes and Complications

Index

Copyright Permission

a CORE Curriculum for Diabetes Education, 5th Edition
American Association of Diabetes Educators

Contact: AADE, 800/338-3633; fax 312/424-2427; e-mail:

The information contained in a CORE Curriculum for Diabetes Education, 5th Edition, is based on the collective experience of the diabetes educators who assisted in its production. Reasonable steps have been taken to make it as accurate as possible based on published evidence as of June 2003. But the Association cannot warrant the safety or efficacy of any product or procedure described in a CORE Curriculum for Diabetes Education, 5th Edition, for application in specific cases. Individuals are advised to consult an appropriate healthcare professional before undertaking any diet or exercise program or taking any medication referred to in a CORE Curriculum for Diabetes Education, 5th Edition. Healthcare professionals must use their own professional judgment, experience, and training in applying the information contained herein. The American Association of Diabetes Educators and its officers, directors, employees, agents, and members assume no liability whatsoever for any personal or other injury, loss, or damages that may result from use of a CORE Curriculum for Diabetes Education, 5th Edition.

TO WHOM IT MAY CONCERN:
Permission is hereby granted from the American Association of Diabetes Educators under the following terms:

ISSN/ISBN #1-881876-15-2

Book Title: _____

Chapter Title: _____

Page Numbers: _____

Permission Granted To: _____

Permission is granted for one-time use only and for educational purposes only.

Complete credit line should appear on all reproductions as follows:
"Reprinted with permission from A Core Curriculum for Diabetes Education, copyright _____, the American Association of Diabetes Educators."

_____   _____
AADE PUBLISHER   DATE